Language Learning and the Brain

Every person who encounters or learns another language is faced with the challenge of processing many new words in a short period of time. What are the conditions under which a learner can acquire those words successfully and process them to long-term memory? How do language and memory faculties interact? What role do the senses play in this process? Are factors such as age or individual backgrounds of learners to be considered? Taking the reader on a fascinating journey through the brain to demonstrate how language is processed, Ulf Schütze explains the dynamic environment involved in recording and producing words. The book also discusses how to use information technology, such as apps, to make the learning of words entertaining and efficient.

ULF SCHÜTZE is an Associate Professor of Second Language Acquisition in the Department of Germanic & Slavic Studies at the University of Victoria, Canada. His research in computer-assisted language learning, lexical processing, as well as the sustainability of technology in second language acquisition has been published in journals worldwide.

Language Learning and the Brain

Lexical Processing in Second Language Acquisition

Ulf Schütze

University of Victoria

CAMBRIDGE
UNIVERSITY PRESS

CAMBRIDGE
UNIVERSITY PRESS

University Printing House, Cambridge CB2 8BS, United Kingdom

Cambridge University Press is part of the University of Cambridge.

It furthers the University's mission by disseminating knowledge in the pursuit of education, learning and research at the highest international levels of excellence.

www.cambridge.org
Information on this title: www.cambridge.org/9781107158450

First published 2017

A catalogue record for this publication is available from the British Library

Library of Congress Cataloging-in-Publication data
Names: Schütze, Ulf, author.
Title: Language learning and the brain : lexical processing in second language acquisition / Ulf Schütze.
Description: Cambridge, United Kingdom : Cambridge University Press, [2016] | Includes bibliographical references and index.
Identifiers: LCCN 2016026222 | ISBN 9781107158450 (hardback : alk. paper)
Subjects: LCSH: Second language acquisition–Psychological aspects. | Language acquisition–Psychological aspects. | Lexicology–Psychological aspects. | Cognitive learning. | Brain–Physiology. | Psycholinguistics. | Neurolinguistics.
Classification: LCC P118.2 .S386 2016 | DDC 401/.93–dc23
LC record available at https://lccn.loc.gov/2016026222

ISBN 978-1-107-15845-0 Hardback

Für Anne und Albrecht

Contents

List of Figures

Preface

Every person learning another language is faced with the challenging task of learning many new words in a short period of time. Much of the success of learning another language depends on what our brain can handle at a time, also known as the cognitive load. The question is, under what conditions a learner can indeed acquire those words, remember and use them when speaking another language. For example, how do language and memory faculties interact? What role do the senses play in this process? Are factors such as age or individual backgrounds of learners to be considered? Taking the reader on a journey through the brain from a psycholinguistic point of view, this book focuses on explaining the dynamics of creating a record of a word using synapses, the hippocampus, the phonological loop, and other areas of the brain. Particular attention is given to spacing techniques and their development and improvement by using information technology, in order that the next app on a smartphone will make the learning of words entertaining and efficient.

Introduction

This book describes how a word is processed when encountered for the first time, in particular if that word is from another language. We encounter other languages in our lives more than we think; for example, in our hometown while shopping for groceries at the supermarket or when watching a foreign film with subtitles. In this book, I will refer to other or second languages as L2 and our first language as L1. For most of us, there was one L1 when we grew up. However, some children have parents who speak different first languages or grow up in a country where the language predominantly spoken is different than those of their parents. In such situations it is sometimes difficult to determine which is the L1 and which is the L2. It depends on the amount of contact a child has with each language. Some children grow up bilingual; that is, they learn two languages at the same time. The question, then, is if the two languages are equal or if one is favored over the other.

Many factors influence how we learn another language. The age at the time of acquisition plays a role, as does the type of environment, the language in which it is encountered, our individual background (knowledge of our first or other languages; analytical, creative, and/or social skills) and motivation to learn that language, and how all of this develops over time. Another factor that has to be considered but is often neglected is how much information our brain can actually handle when processing language (Robinson, 2003; Skehan, 1998, 2009a). This is often referred to as the cognitive load. Every person who encounters or learns another language is faced with the challenge of acquiring many new words in a short period of time. Most languages have a repertoire of 100,000 words or more, although a vocabulary of about 5,000 words is sufficient to communicate in another language in most situations (Schmitt, 2010b). One line of research is to investigate under what conditions an adult learner can:

- acquire those words
- process those words to long-term memory
- recall words when needed
- utter the recalled words.

Studies in cognitive psychology have shown that, in order to process words to long-term memory, spacing techniques work well; that is, to repeat words within a certain time frame. These techniques can be used to acquire a word within the same learning session, which lasts from seconds to minutes, or over multiple learning sessions. In a multiple learning session a word is rehearsed on day one and recalled in another learning session on the following day, or days later. Studies in cognitive psychology have investigated word acquisition within one learning session, although there have been exceptions (for an overview, see Balota, Duchek, and Logan, 2007. This will be discussed in detail in Chapter 7, "Spacing"). In the attempt to learn another language, however, we often find that the word just learned in one session is quickly forgotten in the next. Research in this area therefore looks at how words can be retained over the long term, and what can be done in two or more learning sessions to ensure that they can indeed be recalled. Regardless of whether we aim to investigate one or more learning sessions, the questions are:

- How often does a word need to be repeated?
- What type of repetition (interval) needs to be used?
- What is the time frame (for acquisition)?

To remember a word in the long term means to be able to recall it weeks and months later. It is important to distinguish long-term from short-term gains in memory, an issue that until recently has been blurred. If we use a certain technique to learn words now and are able to recall them tomorrow, does it follow that we can recall the same words a month from now? Or do we need to use a different technique? These are questions that second language specialists try to answer. Several studies have been carried out over many years in the area of lexical processing, which is how single words are recognized, and lexical production, which is how single words are recalled. This includes some of my research, which involves the collection of data from hundreds of university students in an attempt to distinguish between the recognition and recall processes. As we have reached a point in time where results from studies of different disciplines such as cognitive psychology and second language acquisition reach similar conclusions, some cross-disciplinary findings will be presented here.

In addition, I will discuss word groups in further detail. A general problem with studies in second language vocabulary learning is that a distinction between word groups is seldom made. In textbooks, dictionaries, and online programs, all words are treated the same. One simply has to read the newspaper – either in paper format or on a smartphone or tablet – to realize that some words are more difficult to pronounce than others. Pronunciation is a key factor when processing words. For example, much is currently written on the brain, using such words as "hippocampus" or "amygdala." These words are not easy to remember, because they consist of several syllables. In the case of "amygdala," the syllables are also difficult to pronounce. This same pronunciation problem often occurs when we learn words from another language. Longer words are more difficult, because the brain has more syllables to process, but not necessarily any more time to do so than when it processes a shorter word. Another factor is phonological similarity. If a word in two languages is similar in meaning and form, then it is readily acquired in the language to be learned. However, if two or more words in the language to be learned are similar in sound, the brain will need extra time to discriminate their sounds from their meaning. This, of course, makes the learning process longer and more difficult. Somewhat related to phonological similarity is the fact that words with irregular or unexpected sound combinations are also more difficult to process. For example, the English words "plough" and "through" are pronounced differently, even though the combination of vowels and consonants in "-ough" is the same. Since the phonemes of these words do not follow a regular pattern, they require more time to be identified. Such words, then, are more difficult for the English-language learner to acquire.

With regards to processing words, the importance of such criteria as word length and phonological similarity has been researched and understood in cognitive psychology since the 1960s (Baddeley, 2007). Unfortunately, these findings have not been applied to learning new words in another language. The late 1960s through early 1990s was a period of grammar-focused research in second language acquisition. The learning of words – vocabulary acquisition – was set aside, yet no grammar in the world will enable us to communicate. Historically, it is worth noting that in the early 1960s, prior to the grammar craze, there was a significant amount of interest in word research, including lexical processes. When word-focused research made a comeback in the late 1980s and early 1990s, much of it was vocabulary driven; that is, focusing on how to learn words from a pedagogical perspective, in interactions between learners and/or between learners and learning material (Zimmerman, 2009). The study of vocabulary acquisition was informed by the experience of language instructors, which led to the development of methods such as word association, word-trees, and mind-maps (Meara, 2009). However, some researchers did focus on word acquisition (Ellis, 1996; Hulstijn and Laufer, 2001; Webb, 2005) rather than word use. These studies collected large data sets and used inferential statistics to analyze the data. The subjects in these studies were often undergraduate students learning another language. Recently, studies in second language vocabulary acquisition have gone a step farther by investigating lexical processing when the brain encounters a new word (Schütze, 2015). These investigations focus on the word itself, breaking it down into the smallest units: lexemes and phonemes. They also consider linguistic and non-linguistic factors that contribute to a word's successful, long-term memory storage, and its retrieval. The aim of those studies is to focus on how words are processed in the brain before drawing conclusions on how the learners' knowledge can be utilized (Milton, 2009; Nation, 2001). In order to know how to use a word, we have to understand how the record of the word was first created. A word can only be recalled if it has first been successfully stored.

As mentioned, it is helpful to investigate factors related to processing difficulty (length, phonological similarity) when researching second language vocabulary acquisition. In addition to these linguistic elements, we also need to consider a non-linguistic factor: emotional connotation. To understand how emotions affect language acquisition, let's use the words from the example above, the "hippocampus" and the "amygdala." Both are two key brain regions involved in word acquisition. The hippocampus is an area deep down in the brain where the record of a word is created. The amygdala consists of groups of nuclei right next to the hippocampus and is responsible for processing emotion. When a record of a word is created in the hippocampus, not only are language and memory faculties involved but also the senses. Neurotransmitters such as serotonin, dopamine, and acetylcholine play a role when processing emotion, as well as in the formation of new synapses that are needed to solidify the record of a word. One question is whether words with an emotional connotation can be fast-tracked, because when the senses are heightened such sensory information adheres to the brain's record of the word, which could result in a stronger, longer-lasting registry. Interestingly enough, this phenomenon has not been studied when acquiring words in another language. Another question asks whether, due to higher levels of estrogen, which stimulate serotonin, women have a natural advantage when learning words in another language. These and other questions will be discussed in more detail in Chapters 3 and 8, "Synaptic Connections" and "Word Analysis."

In conclusion, in terms of processing, it is useful to distinguish words by groups, including:

- number of syllables (word length)
- similarity
  - meaning (lexemes)
  - pronunciation (phonemes)
  - both (lexemes and phonemes)
- emotional connotations/situations (emotional words).

Research into lexical processing and production is carried out in a variety of disciplines. To understand how a second language is acquired and spoken, we first need to understand the biochemical processes that occur when the brain transmits, stores, and recalls information. Studies in neurophysiology seem to have narrowed down how that happens (for an overview, see Kandel, 2006); however, we also need to test how different parts of the brain operate in the facilitation of lexical processing and production. For decades, studies in cognitive psychology tried to explain the role of language faculties in the brain in conjunction with those associated with memory. With regard to rehearsing and repeating words, there seems finally to be some agreement as to what factors play a role and how they influence the outcome of whether a word is successfully processed and, if so, for how long (for an overview, see Baddeley, Eysenck, and Anderson, 2009). In second language acquisition, we need to consider that the primary reason to learn another language is communication. Our ability to process words to long-term memory is therefore only the first step, as we must also be able to recall words and to use them when needed. Thus, we need to investigate comprehension as well as production (for an overview, see Skehan, 1998). Possible collaborations in research across various disciplines might look like this:

- biological foundation: neurophysiology
- methods: cognitive psychology
- experience: second language learning.

In the last few years, the methods of cognitive psychology have found their way into second language research, thereby informing the learning and teaching of second language acquisition. At the same time, neuroscientists have begun using neuroimaging to monitor a participant's brain as s/he processes another language. Much more such interdisciplinary research must be carried out, especially since the results of such studies are beginning to overlap or to suggest similar direction. The emerging picture of second language processes and acquisition still needs to be refined through the cooperation of neuroscientists, cognitive psychologists, and second language specialists. Nevertheless, current technology and research now allow us to draw conclusions as to how to optimize learning new words. At the end of this book, we will look at how new media, in particular numerous online flashcard systems, are used to acquire new words. Some of these systems place an emphasis on the presentation of words through the use of pictures, audio, or sample sentences. Few of these systems pay attention to various spacing techniques, but a distinction between short-term gains and long-term memory is generally not being made. Hardly any of these systems use algorithms to assist learners of another language acquiring new words. In Chapter 9, "Learning and Teaching," we discuss in more detail the development of online applications that take these factors into account.

Furthermore, we should also note the way in which researchers in first and second language acquisition work with a variety of participants to discover precisely what happens when a word is encountered and/or recalled. In general, there are three groups:

1. Research with healthy subjects:
   a. Children who learn another language in childhood.
   b. Young adults who enroll in a program of modern language at college or university.

2. Research with subjects who have a specific language impairment (SLI). These are usually children who have normal cognitive functioning and scores of general intelligence, but problems with speech. Most of those problems can be dealt with and corrected by a university-trained speech therapist.
3. Research with subjects who are affected by injuries or illnesses to the brain:
   a. Injuries, for example, caused by a stroke or car accident.
   b. Illnesses, for example, Down's syndrome (affecting children early on in life) or Alzheimer's (affecting adults later on in life).

Today, all of these disciplines benefit from advances made in technology. The improvement of neuroimaging techniques such as PET (positron emission tomography) scans, fMRI (functional magnetic resonance imaging), MEG (magnetoencephalography), or EEG (electroencephalography) has contributed to our understanding of lexical processing but less so of lexical production. We must interpret the results of studies using such techniques to explain language acquisition with caution. Many regions of the brain are activated when we process and produce a word, not just the ones related to language (Broca's and Wernicke's area, and the phonological loop), but also the limbic system (the hippocampus and amygdala), and various cortices that transmit information from the senses. Therefore, if we only consult computerized brain scans, it can be difficult to determine precisely what occurs when we process a word. We will learn more about these techniques in Chapter 2, "Memory, Language, and the Brain."

In this book, I will describe how we acquire words in another language. This process is dynamic and fluid. It combines language processing faculties such as the phonological loop (that is, part of working memory proposed by Baddeley, 2007; Baddeley and Hitch, 1974), as well as memory faculties such as the hippocampus, plus the senses. This process is linked to spacing techniques; that is, to repeat words in predefined intervals (first tested by Landauer and Bjork, 1978). We will look at this loop – spacing link under the umbrella of the limited capacity model (a theory developed for second language acquisition by Skehan, 2009a) and underlying principles of synapse formation (using Kandel's, 2006) research in neurophysiology). However, the concepts I bring together in this book are not intended to develop a model of sorts. The idea is to accept second language word acquisition for what it is: a multidirectional process where information is exchanged constantly. The idea is also to accept the individuality of the learner/speaker when learning another language at the beginner's level. Furthermore, we need to consider the environment in which we are acquiring the language. With that many variables, we will be hard pressed to compartmentalize this process into a model. So let's begin our journey through the brain on the heels of a word.

1 A New Word

What It Means to Know a Word

Before we can say a word, we need to know the word. Before we access a word, we need to recall it. Before we can recall a word, we need to have encountered and processed it to the extent that we can recognize and bring it forward (from within our memory) for use at a later time. This is a challenging task. Languages such as English and German have more than 100,000 words (although less than 10 percent of those are used in 90 percent of all written or spoken texts). That means they also have about 100,000 lexemes.

There are many aspects to consider when it comes to how we learn a word, and these considerations are part of a multilevel model developed by Nation (2001). An important distinction must be made between the word's form and meaning as opposed to its multiple usages. For the purpose of investigating word processing from first encounter to long-term memory, I will focus on form and meaning. Once we know how a word is processed and retrieved in our brain, we can look at how it is used in various contexts.

With regard to form and meaning, Nation makes the following distinctions:

- the spoken form of the word (form)
- the written form of the word (form)
- the question of what parts of a word are needed in order to recognize or produce a word (form)
- the relationship of form to meaning (meaning)
- the concept the word expresses (meaning)
- the question of what other words the word is associated with (meaning).

Once the aspects of form and meaning are acquired, we need to learn a word's multiple usages (Nation, 2001): the grammatical patterns of a word, collocations, as well as when and how often we encounter or use a particular word.

We can use Nation's model and link it to phonemes (spoken form), lexemes (written form), and lemmas (concept/the question of what other words the word is associated with). Matching phonemes to lexemes represents the form-to-meaning relationship. Morphemes would be linked to the question of what parts of a word are needed in order to recognize or produce a word, as well as to grammatical patterns. As was explained earlier, these are identified/attached after the phonemes and lexemes have been processed, even though morphemes can feed information back to that process. The form-to-meaning relationship can be complex. By drawing on Nation's multilevel model, Schmitt (2010a) points out that we need to be exposed to a word several times in order to fully understand a word's form-to-meaning relationship.

In terms of processing, we distinguish between phonemes, lexemes, morphemes, and graphemes. A phoneme is best described as a speech unit expressing a distinct sound; that is, a sound that is different when compared to another sound. Encountering a new word, a number of phonemes need to be identified. They are grouped as syllables. The correct order of phonemes, as well as the syllables, needs to be established. This is done via nodes that keep information on what is called serial order. We will go into more detail regarding nodes and serial order in Chapter 4, "Cognitive Load."

A lexeme is an abstract unit that describes the form-to-meaning relationship of a single word. A lexeme needs to be identified, in particular, the concept of a lexeme that is expressed through a lemma. A lemma is part of a lexeme. In addition to the lemma, a lexeme includes possible morphological markers that indicate if and what type of morpheme can be attached. A concept, the idea behind a word, can sometimes be difficult to define. Let us think about the word "coffee." We have an idea of what coffee is, but what exactly are its features? It is made from beans that grow on plants. When brewed, it is dark. It is usually hot when consumed, but there are many variations on how to consume it. Other features, such as strength and size of the coffee, may also be noted. If we follow this thought pattern, we find that there are often various exceptions to the features of a concept that at first seemed well defined. The easiest way to define a concept may be simply to accept what has been commonly agreed upon, in this case, the accepted understanding of what "coffee" means. It may help to look up the definition in a dictionary.

The lemma matches the concept onto the lexeme. It is necessary to have the lemma as a mediator because, on the one hand, a concept can be difficult to define and, on the other hand, there can be several ways of grammatically coding a concept, and some of those ways might in turn change the concept. The grammatical coding is done with the help of the lexeme, which contains information in its morphological markers as to if and what type of morphemes may be attached. In a sense, a marker allows an actual morpheme to be attached. Most important for the form of a word are bound morphemes. A bound morpheme is a unit that can change the meaning or the form of the word if added to the lexeme. There are two types of bound morphemes: derivational and inflectional. Derivational morphemes such as "-ness" or "un-" change the meaning ("happy" becomes "happiness" or "unhappy") and inflectional morphemes such as Third

Person Singular (3.P.Sg.) Present Tense "-s" change the form. In this process the marker functions like a placeholder; that is, a bound morpheme can be attached later if it has been marked. With a match, the morpheme is attached to the lexeme. For example, the lexeme "to walk" has the inflectional morphemes "-s" (pronoun-verb agreement), "-ed," and "-ing" (verb tense), changing the word to "walks," "walked," "walking." The rules that govern which morphemes are attached to which words are very strict and depend on other words in the sentence, such as the pronoun (for example, 3.P.Sg "he" or "she").

Research by Myers-Scotton and Jake (2000) has gone into more detail regarding morphemes. They use the term "system morphemes" to refer to a more elaborate version of bound morphemes. They distinguish between three types of system morphemes. First, there are early system morphemes that occur at the lemma level – for example, the plural "-s," as the lemma will match a concept of two or more things and not just one. Second, there are late system morphemes that attach at the grammar level, for example 3.P.Sg. Present Tense "-s": "I walk" vs. "He walks." In this case, the verb "walk" is recalled and processed fully until it is put into a sentence obeying a grammatical rule. Third, there are bridge system morphemes marked at the lemma level but put into form at the grammar level, for example the possessive "-'s," as in "Angie's coffee." This classification is very helpful for predicting the process of second language acquisition. We will return to it in Chapter 6, "The Bilingual Lexicon and Speaker."

In addition to the phonemes, lexemes, and morphemes, there are also graphemes. Graphemes are essentially letters representing the written form of a word. Naturally, graphemes also need to be processed, but their processing is relatively uncomplicated compared to phonemes or lexemes. Children process graphemes later in life than phonemes because, at the age of five or six, they learn to read and write and thereby come to acquire the orthographic form of the thousands of words they already know. Interestingly, although most adults learning another language do so in order to be able to have a conversation in that language, they often learn words by looking at the orthographic form. Much of that has to do with the way words are presented in textbooks or learning programs.

There are two things that are quite interesting about graphemes when, in addition to hearing a new word, it is also spelled out. In the first scenario, the pronunciation follows a regular pattern; for example, the English word "though" with the diphthong [ou] in between consonants on each side. In this case, processing the lexeme and its orthographic form requires little energy and attention. In the second scenario, let us consider the words "through" or "plough" or "enough." Here is the same combination of the diphthong to the consonants, yet the pronunciation is different. In this case, the graphemes have actually interfered with the phonemes, requiring more attention and consequently more energy from the speaker.

This shows how truly complex it is to process phonemes. Regardless of whether the graphemes assist or interfere with processing the diphthong [ou], in each of those words this diphthong plays a central role in relation to the lexeme of the word. This interplay between phonemes and the lexeme is at the heart of word processing. The linguistic record of the word that is created consists of the lemma of the lexeme indicating a concept, the morphological markers, and a tag that indicates the combination of the phonemes to the particular lexeme. The word record also contains other information, such as emotions conveyed through the senses at the time of input. When a speaker needs to use a word, s/he recalls the records of several lexemes as well as many phonemes, and rehearses them in the phonological loop. The concept is expressed through the lemma of the lexeme. The tag assists in the brain's process of matching phonemes to lexemes, which in turn allows the speaker to recall the correct combination. Once recalled and matched correctly, the interaction with morphemes takes place through the morphological marker of the lexeme. If a morpheme that fits is found, the word will be uttered properly. If not, the process of rehearsal might start again.

In summary, the form-to-meaning relationship of a word is made up by phonemes and lexemes. The phonemes represent the sounds. The lexeme with its lemma and markers must be matched to the phonemes in order to identify the meaning of the word. Later, morphemes are analyzed in order to process the form. Similarly, when a word needs to be recalled from memory for use in speech, the phonemes need to be matched to a lexeme while the morpheme in question, one of many, is processed later, when the final form is determined. The final form can depend on other words in the sentence. Therefore, a morpheme feeds information back to the lexeme that has been matched to its phonemes because, if it does not fit, either another morpheme is tried or another lexeme with its phonemes is rehearsed.

All this happens in our brain in hundreds of milliseconds. The processes are multidirectional; that is, they influence each other. Information from morphemes is fed back to lexemes, information from lexemes to phonemes, and from phonemes to morphemes. The details of this process are very intriguing, not all of which have been fully explored or understood. However, many advances have recently been made in the fields of neurophysiology, cognitive psychology, and second language acquisition that provide some insight as to what happens in our brain when we process and speak another language.

First Encounter

It is quite exciting for the brain to learn a new word. Phonemes, lexemes, morphemes, and graphemes are all components of a new word that the brain must analyze. The process of identifying those '–emes' requires the activation of several regions in the brain. Information necessary to process the new word is transported through neuroanatomical circuits that connect language faculties, memory faculties, and emotions via the senses. The brain lights up, so to speak, as neurons fire simultaneously in communication with each other (Singer, 2006). If the process is successful, a synapse is created to connect the neurons (nerve cells able to transmit information) and store the record of the word. These synapses create permanent access to the information in the form of a bridge or path (Kandel, 2006). Yet nothing is permanent when it comes to memory. The strength of the synaptic connection – which we might compare figuratively to a bridge in the form of an eight-lane highway overpass, a rural covered trestle, or a tree trunk over a wilderness creek bed – depends on how the word is encountered. The following factors influence this result:

- situation (modalities: audio, visual, example)
- word group (length, similarity, emotional connotation)
- word category (content vs. function words)
- spacing (uniform vs. expanded)
- timing (number of repetitions, time frame).

Depending on the given situation, a new word can be encountered in spoken conversation; by listening or overhearing other people talking; or by reading, whether in a text on your cell phone, in an email, or in a newspaper or book. In any case, the brain's challenge is to match the phonemes to a lexeme. When talking to someone, the listener relies on audible sounds. When reading, that person must decipher the sounds by looking at the graphemes. Ideally, the learner both hears and reads the word simultaneously, in order to receive both verbal and written information cues. This also depends on the type of learner: some people prefer to hear sounds in order to identify a word, while others require the visual input. Recent studies have shown that non-linguistic information, in particular pictures, plays a key role when processing a new word (Jones and Plass, 2002; Kim and Gilman, 2008). That is, the likelihood of a strong word record is higher when a corresponding image is processed.

Situational factors also refer to where the word is encountered. A major factor is whether or not you are in the country where the language you are learning is predominantly spoken. Imagine you are learning German. In Germany, Austria, or some other parts of Europe where German is spoken, you will not only be surrounded by the sounds of German, you will also pick up extra non-linguistic information beyond the new words, such as the taste and smell of the coffee you drink, the colorful arrangement of tiles on the table at which you sit, and the hairstyle and outfit of the waiter who brings you the coffee. All of these sensory cues are examples of non-linguistic information that may be encoded through cortices in your brain and fed via emotional responses to the hippocampus, in order to strengthen the record of the word. It is difficult to create such a rich, sensory situation when we study a second language within the classroom. Some language programs try to use information technology to immerse the learner into an online environment to compensate for the lack of actually being immersed in the foreign country. The problem is that our brain is capable of processing highly specific nuance, and can determine at once that the locations do not correspond. In such a situation, it is as if our brain could ask: "Why am I sitting in front of a computer and not in a café in Vienna?"

In terms of word groups, it is important to consider the length and similarity of the word encountered. Words with many syllables have many phonemes that need to be identified and matched onto a lexeme. The main problem when processing is the time available to digest the incoming information. In conversation or reading, we encounter many words in a short period of time. All of those, including the ones we know, are rehearsed in the phonological loop (Baddeley, 2007). If a new word is not identified within two seconds, it might not be processed. We will go into more detail in Chapter 4, "Cognitive Load." An additional problem occurs when we encounter words that have similar phonemes because, due to the discrimination process, the brain will need more time to distinguish between the phonemes that overlap. For the success of second language learners, we must account for the predictability of how such phonemes are pronounced. If the word has an unusual pronunciation pattern, a learner needs to rehearse it more often. Sometimes, similarity across languages can be an advantage to the language learner. If words in both the native tongue and the language to be acquired have similar lexemes, the brain will match the new lexeme to the existing with greater ease.

When analyzing word groups, we should also consider the phenomenon of words that have an emotional connotation, such as "love," "cry," or "happy." This emotional information – which is fed through cortices connecting the senses to the hippocampus – is stored in long-term memory along with the lexemes of those words. This creates a strong connection through the synapse. The record will be even more powerful if an emotional word is learned in an emotional situation. For example, if you fall off your bicycle while vacationing in the Rhine Valley, the German word for "to hurt" [verletzen], will be more easily remembered.

Another distinction, in terms of processing, can be made between content and function words. The criteria to distinguish between word groups – length, similarity, emotional connotation – mostly apply to content words such as nouns, verbs, adjectives, and some adverbs. These words have an independent meaning. Other types of words, called function words, such as prepositions, conjunctions, fillers, and some adverbs, carry meaning only in connection with content words. For example, imagine you order a coffee with milk. You know what "coffee" is, but what is the preposition "with"? Meaning is only assigned by asking "with what?" In other words, "with milk." In any language, there are few function words compared to the number of content words. In general, function words tend to be short, having three syllables or less. The likelihood of their similarity is not high, as they are few in number. Naturally, function words do not have an emotional connotation, because they do not have independent meaning. This poses an interesting question: does the fact that a function word is short and not similar to another function word indicate that it can be readily processed to long-term memory, or does the fact that it lacks independent meaning – that is, the lexeme is weak – indicate that it needs to be rehearsed often? In research on second language acquisition, this question has only been investigated recently (Schütze, 2015). We will return to this in Chapter 8, "Word Analysis."

We have known for some time that processing is linked to spacing – the repetition of certain words at certain intervals. Spacing, in turn, can be linked to working memory. We will learn more about working memory in the following chapter, "Memory, Language, and the Brain." Research testing different spacing techniques has been carried out since the 1970s (for an overview, see Balota, Duchek, and Logan, 2007). It has been shown that, in order to recall a word successfully, that word must be repeated several times with an intermittent pause between the repetitions. This pause gives the phonological loop a chance to process the word, while it allows the hippocampus to create a record of that word. However, there has been some controversy with regard to the ideal duration of these pauses. For example, should a word be repeated using a uniform interval (repeat – pause – repeat – pause – repeat), or an expanded interval (repeat – repeat – pause – repeat – pause – pause – pause – repeat)? Also related to the question of the ideal type of spacing is the question of timing. Should a new word be acquired in one learning session, where the word is repeated after seconds or minutes, or from one learning session to the next? Or should a word be learned through the process of repetition over a whole day or several days? How many times does a word need to be repeated? This is something cognitive psychologists as well as second language specialists continue to investigate, but the goal of the learner is commonly overlooked. Is the word acquired to be used right away (short-term gain) or to be used later on, whenever needed (long-term memory)? Ideally, it is acquired for both scenarios. However, this can present complications (Roediger and Karpicke, 2010; Schütze and Weimer-Stuckmann, 2011), as we will see in Chapter 7, "Spacing."

In summary, the strength of the synapse depends on the learning situation, word group and category, spacing interval, and overall timing. Synapses form connections that bring pieces of information together across several brain regions. Some such pieces serve language processing and production, such as the phonological loop, Wernicke's area, and Broca's area. Some pieces serve to process sensory information through the cortices and the amygdala, while some pieces, such as the hippocampus, serve to assist with memory. From a psycholinguistic point of view, a new word has been successfully identified when it reaches the hippocampus: a deep, well-protected brain region that creates a record of the word and stores it in the adjacent non-mesial region. We will go into more detail on the brain in Chapter 3, "Synaptic Connections."

Maintenance of a Word

Each time we encounter a word – either new or familiar – and each time we say a word, it is rehearsed in the phonological loop within Broca's area. Back in the early 1970s, when research on the phonological loop was in its infancy, Craik and Lockhart (1972) proposed two types of rehearsal: maintenance rehearsal and elaborate rehearsal. Maintenance rehearsal refers to the simple maintenance of words already known; for example, the repetition of a word, like a street name, to oneself in order not to forget. In contrast, elaborate rehearsal refers to the recitation of new words. In this case the brain must process new information, such as phonemes and lexemes, in connection with other sensory-emotional data in order to create a new word record.

The maintenance of a word should not be underestimated. We need to use it often enough to refresh our memory and to reinforce the synapse-bridge created at the time of recording a word. Any bridge, without proper maintenance, will eventually crumble. Researchers debate the length of time a word record can be stored in our long-term memory. If we attempt to recall a word that has not been thought of for some time, at what point will the attempt fail? The answer depends on how the record of the word was created. If the record is strong, it can be recalled even years later. The strength of the record depends:

- on the type of information recorded; for example, to what degree the senses were activated, and
- on how the word was encountered; for example, if the learner used spacing techniques for repetition.

How does all this play out when learning another language? In first language acquisition, the process of identifying phonemes, lexemes, and lemmas, via the form-to-meaning relationship, is largely automatic. The first few thousand words are learned around the age of three. A native speaker has the full repertoire of phonemes at her or his disposal. A large number of concepts have been developed to help identify the lemma. The rules of morphology to grammatically code a word are learned as early as age three and should be automatic by the age of six to eight.

In second language acquisition, however, the process differs according to the learner's phase of development. Ideally, another language is acquired in childhood, when the development of L1 and L2 go hand in hand. However, most of us learn a second language after the age of six, which means when we go through the language-development phases all the way to the mid-twenties, only some will overlap between L1 and L2. We will discuss this in more detail in Chapter 5, "First and Second Language Acquisition." Let us keep in mind that learning another language is an ongoing process, as Singleton (1995, 2007) points out. Each phase is as important as the one before. For a learner who first encounters the new language at age six, one of the next phases occurs around age eight, when children develop strategies to infer meaning from a word. This widens around the age of twelve or thirteen, when we begin to develop concepts of an abstract nature. Consequently, lemmas change and influence the formation of lexemes. On the plus side, children who learn a language after the age of six to eight have already acquired substantial grammar skills. To acquire grammar rules in another language, although very different than those of the first language, is relatively uncomplicated because we have a general knowledge of how grammar works. With regard to morphemes, sometimes there is a problem in that the L2 morphemes interfere with the L1 morphemes. For example, German verbs add a late system morpheme for every person in Present Tense (First Person Singular to Third Person Plural), not just Third Person Singular, as with English. Beginning German-language students who are native English speakers therefore often forget to add the late system morpheme. While it is not complicated to add morphemes, it must nevertheless be remembered, in particular since late system morphemes already come late to the process of rehearsal in the phonological loop. Some workings of the loop are not refined until about sixteen years of age, which marks another phase.

Naturally, the biggest challenge for an adult language learner is vocabulary: how to remember the multitude of new words? But learning another language successfully should be possible even if that language is not encountered as a child or youth, since the hippocampus, responsible for creating a record of a new word, develops its full potential well into our mid-twenties (Korte, 2009). This is important for university students who enroll in beginners' German, Spanish, and other language courses. Although it might take more effort and time to process thousands of new words, it is possible to learn a language in one's early twenties. We will return to learning words throughout life in Chapter 5, "First and Second Language Acquisition."

In second language acquisition, much of processing words depends on the environment in which these words are encountered. The host country of any language provides more opportunity to process words along with sensory information, as well as to encounter them frequently in order to build and maintain a strong record. Immersion in the L2 environment also assists pronunciation, as the learner is able to hear native pronunciation and prosody (stress, rhythm, intonation). Children develop a repertoire of phonemes in the first year of life and continue to constantly practice pronunciation. By the time they come to school, most children have generally refined their pronunciation of familiar words, though they still make mistakes with new words, especially those that have an unusual pattern of syllables. A child growing up in England with English as his or her L1 will very likely mispronounce the word "plough" the first time s/he reads it aloud. However, once s/he hears the correct pronunciation, s/he will be able to repeat it quickly. If the child learns another language after the age of six to eight, it will take additional time to get the pronunciation right. S/he must not only identify the phonemes, but must also learn the prosody of the word, and train her or his vocal cords and tongue to reproduce those sounds. For most of us, the older we are, the longer it will take to achieve correct pronunciation. There are exceptions, such as with people who have a good ear, like musicians, because they are able to hear the differences between phonemes in L1 and phonemes in L2. Again, a short cut to a good pronunciation is to be in the country where the language is predominantly spoken, as this increases one's opportunity to hear many variations of the word. This in turn helps to fine-tune the ear.

In order to get an idea of how complex it is to process words, as well as of the differences between two languages, Figure 1 shows what is involved when a word is processed in English as well as in German.

All of the linguistic features – phonemes, lexemes, morphemes, graphemes – need to be processed for each word. While there can be agreement in

	phonenes	lexeme/compounds	morphemes	graphemes	other info	word type
to run	[' rʌn]	run/runaway	-s -ing	r-u-n	ran – run (irregular)	verb
laufen	[' laufn]	lauf/Laufweg	-e/-st/-t/-en	l-a-u-f-e-n	lief - gelaufen (irregular)	verb
the chair	[' tʃ eə]	chair/chairlift	-s	c-h-a-i-r	sitting chair head of a committee	noun
der Stuhl	[ʃ tu:1]	Stuhl/Lehrstuhl	-e plus vowel change: ü	S-t-u-h-l	sitting chair stool (med)	noun
crazy	[' kreɪ zɪ]	crazy	-	c-r-a-z-y	craziness	adjective
verrückt	[fɛɐ ' ry kt]	verrückt	- (behind noun) - e/ -en/ -er/ -es - em (before noun)	v-e-r-r-ü-c-k-t	Verrücktheit	adjective

Figure 1. Word Complexity English/German.

the lexemes of two languages – "to run" and "laufen" refer to the same activity; "the chair" and "der Stuhl" refer to the same object; "crazy" and "verrückt" refer to the same emotional state – the phonemes that need to be matched to the lexemes are different. However, subtle differences exist as well: the lexeme of "laufen" does not include the "-en" ending in German, as that is not part of the stem of the verb. Often, compounds are also different. For example, a "Laufweg" is a trail and a "Lehrstuhl" is a professorship. In general, it is possible to create many more compounds in German than in English. The most differences between languages are usually found in morphemes. In German, there are more morphemes than in English: four different types of morphemes in German present tense vs. two morphemes in English present tense; eight ways of forming the plural of nouns in German plus some exceptions vs. two ways of forming the plural in English; and six different morphemes for German adjectives vs. the null-morpheme for English adjectives. The conjugation of verbs can be irregular, thereby changing the lexeme. The meaning of words, of nouns in particular, can be multiple and varied among different languages: "head of a committee" vs. "stool." Adjectives can be turned into nouns: "craziness" and "Verrücktheit." All of these things must be processed in the brain when a new word is encountered. Our brain operates on the principle of efficiency, which breaks a word into parts to record, reassemble, and recall from memory, rather than storing it intact with all its information. We will go into more detail how the brain disassembles, stores, and recalls words in Chapter 2, "Memory, Language, and the Brain."

There is an interesting phenomenon that occurs when we encounter a new word in another language. If that word sounds similar to a word we already know in our first language and has a similar meaning and form, the process of creating a record of that word is fast-tracked because the alignment of its phonemes and lexemes can be matched to an alignment of phonemes and lexemes in our memory that has been created before. These types of words are called cognates. For example, "to sing" in German is "singen"; thus the two languages seem to share a word. However, the difference in pronunciation can sometimes present a problem. While the "s" in "to sing" is pronounced [s], the "s" in "singen" is pronounced [z]. Cognates also occur in some variation. For example, a learner who hears the word "Buch" in German can probably determine that it means "book."

To try to learn several aurally similar words of the same language at once, all of them new and unknown, is not necessarily a good idea. This technique is sometimes used in schools, textbooks, or learning programs to encourage students to remember as many words as possible. This presents two problems. The first involves the cognitive load, which says that our mind can only process so many words at a time. The second problem occurs when we try to choose between too many words with similar phonemes. An excess of similar phonemes will not give the brain enough time to discriminate between them. This happens not only when learning another language but also in a first language. As early as 1966, Baddely has shown that for native speakers of English a word list such as "cat, map, man, cat, mad" is more difficult than word lists such as "pit, day, cow, pen, hot" (examples taken from Baddeley, 1966). This circumstance is known as the phonological similarity effect. The effect disappears when words are repeated several times because each rehearsal adds to the ratio of phonemes discriminated, until with enough repetitions the process is complete. Yet when learning a new language we should avoid making overly long word lists, especially if the words are homonyms.

The example of Figure 1 shows content words: verbs, nouns, adjectives (and some adverbs), as well as all linguistic information processed for those words. We must keep in mind that the record of the word also includes non-linguistic information transmitted by the senses. Another word category is function words: prepositions, conjunctions, some adverbs, and particles. Function words are short and have less information to process. Their lexemes do not have independent meaning. Words such as "very," "with," or "because" only make sense in conjunction with other words. Most notably, they do not have morphemes. The question, then, is whether or not they are processed faster or if they need to be rehearsed more often in the phonological loop, since the lack of information makes it more difficult to discriminate between them. Just as it is possible that too much information complicates the brain's ability to process words within a short period of time, it may also be possible that there is too little. This is a question asked earlier in this chapter, and to which we will return in Chapter 8, "Word Analysis."

Speech Production

There is more to the act of word acquisition than just the components of phonemes, lexemes, morphemes, and graphemes described by cognitive psychologists and linguists. A word also has a lemma that links the lexeme to a concept. Concepts can vary remarkably from language to language as well as being able to overlap.

Imagine you have just arrived in Germany. Still at the airport, you want to drink a coffee. You take out your pocket English-German/German-English dictionary and look up the word "der Kaffee." You find a coffee shop and stand in line. Actually, most likely there will not be a line, as people in Germany tend to go directly to the counter, even if it is crowded. You say, "der Kaffee!" and might earn some funny looks because that actually means, "the coffee!" and not "a coffee." Despite all this, you are able to convey your request. But more surprises are to come. First, "ein Kaffee" comes in a cup so small you wonder if you may have ordered a child's size. Second, the first sip of the coffee tastes unusually strong. You wonder if you actually said "Kaffee" and not "espresso." Now you know that the coffee is smaller in size because it is higher in caffeine. Even with a child's size, your heart rate is racing like it wants to win at Ascot. So, as it turns out, the concept of a "coffee" does not really match the concept of a "Kaffee."

In the above circumstance, all this may become further compounded if we tried to explain to the person who sold us the coffee that the coffee is very strong. Even if we even have the ability to say so in German – "Der Kaffee ist aber stark!" – that person might not understand, since the strength and size of the coffee is normal to her or him. While we learn new words in order to communicate to someone in another language, the key to this successful communication is that we know the words as well as the concepts behind them. Importantly, the person with whom we wish to communicate must also share (or at least understand) these same words and concepts. This is how speaking another language can become so complex and exciting. To put this process in a visual format, see Figure 2.

A conversation starts with the speaker, in this case person 1. Person 1 needs to locate the words s/he wants to use from memory, and then put them into a grammatically correct sentence. Once s/he accomplishes this (pre-utterance sentence), s/he can then choose a medium for the type of communication. For example, if the speaker wants to send a written communication, s/he could tap out a text message. The other person, person 2, in this case the receiver, then has to read the message and decipher the words by accessing his or her word and grammar comprehension. When s/he is ready to respond, person 2 becomes the speaker and must again access his or her word bank in order to find appropriate choices and to grammatically encode them. Now let us imagine that s/he decides to respond by phone call (speaking). When person 1 (now listener) answers the call, s/he must hear and decipher the words, again through the memory, vocabulary, and grammar access. This process goes back and forth in the communication cycle.

At the center of this process are vocabulary and grammar. Whether speaking or writing, the aim is fluent, accurate, and complex communication (Skehan, 1998; Skehan and Foster, 1997). Fluency of speech is linked to the speed with which we can recall words from memory, whereas speaking accurately refers to being able to recall words correctly as well as to grammatically code them with morphemes. Complexity refers to our access to a large variety of words stored in the non-mesial region. This includes those with multiple meanings and therefore highly complex lexemes that correspond to the formation of complex grammatical sentences. We discuss this in more detail in Chapter 4, "Cognitive Load."

Over the years, several models have been developed that attempt to explain speech production. In first language acquisition (L1), Levelt (1989, 1992,

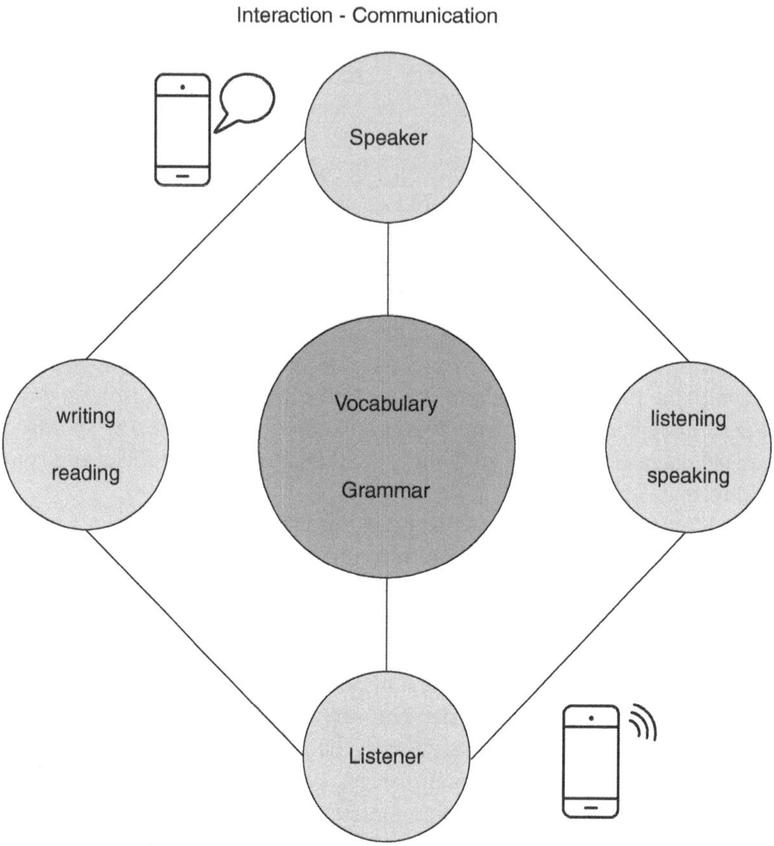

Figure 2. Interaction – Communication.

revised: Levelt, Roelofs, and Meyer, 1999) used different components in his model to break down the process of generating a word. That model has three stages: conceptualization, formulation, and articulation. First, a concept is matched onto the lemma part of the lexeme. Second, in the formulation stage, the lexeme is grammatically coded through a process that identifies the morpheme(s) it requires and its position in the sentence. Following this, the phonemes are matched to the lexeme while the phonemes feed information back to the morpheme(s). Eventually the overall plan is checked in order to confirm the speaker's word choice and to allow her or him to pronounce it. Third, the word/sentence is articulated. Once the word has been spoken, it is checked by a speech comprehension system that monitors all words generated by the speaker, as well as words heard from other speakers.

A general problem with any model is that it is two-dimensional, using boxes and arrows in an attempt to explain a process that is fluid and dynamic. Although most speech comprehension and speech production models point out that the components work simultaneously so various parts of the same sentence are at different processing stages at the same time, the dimension of time is not well represented. It is difficult to use a model to overcome its linearity: A triggers B, B contacts D if A is linked to D with the help of C. In our brain several processes are at work in parallel. When information is transmitted, several brain regions activate simultaneously while language circuits spring into action, forming a network, as Pulvermüller and his team have proposed (Garagnani, Wennekers, and Pulvermüller, 2006; Pulvermüller, 1996). In all, many thousands of neurons fire to process a word.

A particular problem with Levelt's (1989, 1992) model is that grammatical encoding takes place before phonological encoding. In the revised version, Levelt, Roelofs, and Meyer (1999) place more emphasis on the interactivity of grammatical and phonological encoding. Nevertheless, we need to acknowledge that rehearsing lexemes to phonemes in order to identify and match them is the starting point of processing a new word when it is first encountered (speech comprehension), as well as when recalling the record of a word from memory to be used in a sentence (speech production). We will go into more specific detail regarding the rehearsal and matching process of lexemes and phonemes throughout this book. A strong point of Levelt's model, however, is that the dual approach of a speech production (encoding speech: speaking, writing) and speech comprehension (decoding speech: listening, reading) system is particularly evident.

We all know that listening to a song is easier than singing a song. The experience is rather the same when we learn new words: to listen to a new word is easier than recalling and speaking a new word. We usually encounter a new word in the context of a sentence. We hopefully know all the other words in the sentence, which can help us to narrow down the new word's meaning. Yet, before we can use the word correctly in a sentence, we will first need to have learned what it means. Of course, we can just repeat a sentence or imitate the word without its meaning. This is what children do when they are first acquiring a language between the ages of two and three. To speak a word we must also activate our voice in order to pronounce it correctly. As in singing, this can be trained with practice. To learn words in another language, we need to practice the pronunciation of those words.

The difference between production and comprehension is something we need to keep in mind when reviewing experiments that test participants' language skills. Many experiments test comprehension; in particular, those experiments that use neuroimaging techniques. The problem is that, with regard to language, there is always the chance that movement of the jaw will distort images of the brain during the use of scans.

The next question is how speech comprehension and speech production work in second language acquisition (L2). There are more models. Some researchers used Levelt's model, while some developed their own. We will discuss these models in more detail in Chapter 6, "The Bilingual Lexicon and Speaker." Most models attempt to explain speech production in L2 by providing examples of highly proficient bilingual speakers (for an overview, see Kroll and Dijkstra, 2010). These models focus on conceptualizations attempting to determine under what conditions lemmas are transferred from L1 to L2. As regards the formulation stage, morphemes and phonemes are language-specific. We need to learn the grammatical rules of another language (for an overview on different types of morphemes and how they vary among languages, see Myers-Scotton, 2003; Myers-Scotton and Jake, 2000), as well the pronunciation of its phonemes (for an overview on second language phonology, see Archibald, 1998). Therefore, identifying lemmas in another language (or transferring them from L1), encoding morphemes in L2 (recalling grammatical rules), and pronouncing a word (with phonemes that are different in L2 than in L1) places a high demand on our cognitive resources.

One of the central questions in second language acquisition is how much information is transferred and at what level. Generally, it is agreed that the same lemma can be accessed and shared by two or more languages if the concept of the word in L2 is similar to the concept of a word in L1. On the other hand, languages do not share grammatical information coded in morphemes. Morphemes are usually unique to a language. This raises the interesting question as to how a lexeme is accessed in L2, as one part of a lexeme is the lemma and another part of the lexeme is a morphological marker to place a morpheme. In order to solve this puzzle, it is helpful to know that, when we speak a word in either L1 or L2, many lexemes as well as phonemes can be activated, with morphemes activated to a lesser degree. Phonemes are rehearsed in the phonological loop, a part of Broca's area (speech production), until an acceptable combination is found that can be matched onto a lexeme. Rather than asking how a lexeme is accessed, we need to ask how the matching process functions, since many lexemes are activated simultaneously. If we know more than one language, those activated lexemes can be L1 lexemes as well as L2 lexemes, although one of those lexemes will be activated more than the others during the matching process. The likelihood of activation depends on how the record of the word was created when the word was first encountered and processed. We will go into more specific detail regarding the matching process throughout the book. In general, however, the record of a word contains its lexeme (the lemma expressing the concept as well as the morphological marker), a tag that indicates possible combinations of phonemes that can be matched with this lexeme, as well as information transmitted through the senses. If the word is first encountered in written form, the lexeme includes information on spelling by tagging graphemes. Although the lexeme has a marker to place a morpheme, the actual morpheme is not part of the record. In the end, the lexeme chosen is the one activated more than the others. Therefore, all the information that is part of the record of a word plays a role when generating a lexeme, regardless of L1 or L2.

Once phonemes and lexemes are matched and morphemes selected, the word must still be pronounced. Depending on the language, this is not as easy as it sounds. The number of phonemes is actually quite limited. English – which may refer to British English, American English, or Australian English – has between 36 and 48 phonemes and 7 to 10 diphthongs, while standard German has 42 phonemes and 3 diphthongs. Still, the possible combinations seem infinite. As with singing, it is helpful to practice the pronunciation of all those sounds.

Without acquiring words successfully, there is very little we can say. The real question is how that process works in our brain. What does a word consist of? How does the brain transmit the coded information in a word? Under what conditions is the record of a word stored and recalled? How do children, who learn new words every day, process words? How do adults learn another language? What is the difference between L1 and L2? How much information can our memory handle at a time?

To answer these questions, we must analyze words. Naturally, in order to speak another language, it is necessary to build a large vocabulary. In the last twenty or so years, second language researchers have conducted extensive work on word association; that is, how some words can be used to learn other words in order to build a semantic network. Some of that research has looked at different types of texts to find out how often certain words are used and in what way – for example, as part of a phrase. However, we still lack extensive research on single word acquisition. If we want to know how to play with words using associations or how to use words to form a sentence, we must first uncover how the word's smallest units are processed into long-term memory. To this end, research in lexical processing and production must become highly detailed, taking on, for example, the dissection of single words into phonemes, lexemes, graphemes, and morphemes. The smaller the unit we investigate, the more accurate our findings. In order to do so, we must analyze how these '–emes' are processed in the phonological loop and how that relates to other language processing faculties as well as non-linguistic information and memory.

A vocabulary of about 5,000 words is considered sufficient to communicate in another language in most situations (Schmitt, 2010b). There are various opinions on how many words can be acquired per day, ranging from five to twenty (Nation, 2001). If you do the math, acquiring eight words per day translates into acquiring those 5,000 words in less than two years. Most college or university foreign language programs operate on the premise to acquire grammar and vocabulary within two years in order to expand and practice the language in years three and four. Although learning eight words per day does not seem that much, the way our brain processes words indicates that new words need to be repeated several times over several days in order to be stored in long-term memory. The acquisition should be staggered using spacing intervals. In the next chapter, we learn more about working memory, as well as limited attentional capacity, which provides the theoretical framework for processing words. In Chapters 7–9, "Spacing," "Word Analysis," and "Learning and Teaching," we find out about optimal spacing patterns and online programs that assist in acquiring all those words efficiently without overburdening the cognitive load.

2 Memory, Language, and the Brain

Stages of Processing

As noted in the previous chapter, several aspects of form and meaning play a role when acquiring a new word (Nation, 2001). Right from the start, the form-to-meaning relationship needs to be developed. Phonemes and lexemes need to be identified, matched, and the record of this match stored, so when we need to speak the record of the word we are looking for can be called up. There are three stages of word processing: coding, storage, and retrieval. One of the challenges for a learner is processing a word in time. A key component in the brain's process of acquiring new words is working memory (Baddeley, 2007). It serves to prolong the duration of time our brain has to rehearse a word in order to identify its phonemes and lexeme. This increases the likelihood that the brain will create a record of the word that is then stored near the hippocampus in an area called the non-mesial region. If a record is created, the word can be recalled at a later time. The process of creating a record of a word is referred to as "episodic in nature," while recalling a word that has been acquired is "semantic in nature" (Paradis, 1994). Both the episodic and the semantic component are part of declarative knowledge.

When we learn a new language we rely on declarative knowledge. However, when we are young and learn our first language we need another type of knowledge called procedural knowledge. Declarative and procedural knowledge are linked. Procedural knowledge refers to figuring out operational sequences, for example, how to ride a bicycle. In regards to language, a child has to decipher how language works as a system: how to identify phonemes, how to match them to a lexeme, how to grammatically code a word, and how to connect words to form sentences. For children growing up with two languages, the task is a further challenge as they must sort/code the vocabulary and grammar rules of two languages into their developing word process system. Between the ages of three and five, a child will often make errors when it applies the rules of one language to words from the other. Of course, these kinds of errors are also made by adults who learn another language. However, these errors occur less frequently, because as adults we already understand how language works as a system.

Also active when the brain processes phonemes and lexemes are other cognitive functions, such as: attention, which is directed toward the incoming word before it is rehearsed subvocally in the loop; the senses, which feed information perceived while the word was encountered to the hippocampus; and the amygdala, which plays a key role in the brain's emotion processes.

In order to be processed, a word needs to be attended to (Schmidt, 1995, 2001). However, our attentional resources are not endless (Robinson, 2003; Skehan, 2009a). This is the premise of the limited capacity model proposed by Skehan (2009a) and Skehan and Foster (2001). The model focuses on speech production and considers three aspects of speech: linguistic and lexical complexity (variety of grammatical structures and vocabulary); cognitive processing (sufficiency, clarity, and organization of information with regard to the content of the message that is to be produced); and communicative stress (time pressure during interaction, speed, and type of utterance). These aspects compete for attention.

Skehan and Foster (1999) carried out a series of experiments with English as a Foreign Language learners at Thames Valley University whose proficiency level was described as "lower intermediate." The participants watched episodes from the TV series *Mr. Bean* and then had to retell the episode. Results showed that participants who had to retrieve words that are not commonly used spoke at a slower rate, and also made more grammatical mistakes. The attention was on the lexeme, compromising fluency and accuracy. Skehan and Foster argue that second language learners first and foremost aim at reaching the communicative goal, i.e., they will prioritize meaning over form. The attention that is left for form needs to be shared between linguistic complexity, accuracy, and fluency. We will come back to complexity, accuracy, and fluency of speech in Chapter 4, "Cognitive Load." In another study, Skehan (2009b) showed that native speakers do not have to compromise. In fact, using complex lexemes can benefit a native speaker's syntax.

Every time we encounter a word, it needs to be processed. If the word is unfamiliar, it needs to receive enough attention to be rehearsed, matched, and stored. At the forefront of this process is what is known as working memory (Baddeley, 1986, 1999, 2007; Baddeley and Hitch, 1974). Studies have been carried out since the 1960s with healthy learners (often undergraduate students), patients (with an injury or illness affecting memory and language), as well as children with SLI, testing retention or recall of digits, non-words, uncommon words, or natural words. In general, studies revealed that poor phonological memory negatively impacts the acquisition of new words (Gathercole and Baddeley, 1990).

The function of working memory is to prolong the time during which words can be processed. This is a temporary process. The main component is the so-called central executive that directs, divides, and switches attention to incoming words, a process that demands much energy (Baddeley, 2007). As in the limited capacity model, the executive control will direct attention to allocate resources. The central executive is linked to factors such as the learner's motivation, familiarity or unfamiliarity with the word, and the word group (length/similarity/emotional connotation). If the executive control decides that a word is important enough to be processed, words are processed by another device called the phonological loop, which rehearses and temporarily stores the phonemes of those words. This happens subvocally. The loop can code auditory (listening/speaking) as well as visual information (reading/writing). It does so by binding novel sounds into sequences that make up words. The phonemes must be identified by their combination of vowels and consonants, and must also be matched to a lexeme in Wernicke's area. The lexeme's lemma and morphological marker must then be identified. When we learn a new word in another language, sometimes the existing lexeme must be modified, or an entirely new lexeme must be created. The loop has two separate subsystems: rehearsal and temporary storage. They work in parallel. The phonemes of one word (or more) can be rehearsed at the same time as a new word (or more) arrives. If the phonemes are not identified right away, they can be parked in the storage subsystem. If they are identified but cannot be matched to a lexeme in Wernicke's area, they can go back to the loop and be parked again. If many words are rehearsed, need to go back, or come in simultaneously, they compete for attention as they are matched. If a word does not get the attention, it falls out of the loop. If we recognize that we have missed a word, we might ask, "Excuse me, can you repeat that, please?" to start the process of rehearsing that word again. In addition, the word's bound or system morphemes need to be identified, if they are present. That happens at a slightly later stage in Wernicke's area. These processes of phoneme, lexeme, and morpheme identification overlap and go back and forth as they feed information to each other. Usually, we encounter a new word in another language when we hear it in conversation or on the radio or when we read a text message, email, or the newspaper. If we hear a word, the phonemes go directly to the loop and are rehearsed. If we see a word, it must be transcribed into a phonological code before it can be rehearsed. This is an extra step. Once the code has been transcribed, though, the phonemes are processed as usual. In fact, the visual code can assist the brain to match the word's phonemes to its lexemes. This information can become part of the record of a word that is created in the hippocampus.

The process of rehearsal is fragile, as Baddeley, Gathercole, and Papagno (1998) have pointed out. In the loop, either rehearsal or storage can be interrupted, as studies with patients suffering from memory loss have shown. We will discuss those studies in more detail in Chapter 4, "Cognitive Load." Rehearsal takes place in the left prefrontal cortex of the brain and is part of Broca's area, while temporary storage takes place in the left side of the parietal lobe.

Another component of working memory is the so-called visuo-spatial sketchpad that processes non-language information; for example, shapes we see, colors, and location of objects or movement (Baddeley, 2007).

Furthermore, Baddeley (2007) argues that in between the phonological loop and visuo-spatial sketchpad is one more component called the episodic buffer. It has no active role in lexical processing but simply provides a link between the executive, the loop, and the sketchpad. Other than that, little is known about the episodic buffer.

In summary, the three stages of processing are:

1. Coding: When we first encounter a word, the phonemes of the word are rehearsed subvocally in the phonological loop, which has two subsystems: rehearsal and temporary storage. These phonemes are then matched to a lexeme in Wernicke's area of speech comprehension. The phonological loop and Wernicke's area constantly exchange information until a match has been found. Morphemes are identified at a later stage. The word – that is, the combination of the phonemes to the lexeme – is then forwarded to the hippocampus. The hippocampus is where the record of the word, which consists of linguistic and non-linguistic information, is created. The non-linguistic information is transmitted by the senses to the hippocampus, including emotions transmitted by the amygdala.
2. Storage: The record of the word is stored in an area called the non-mesial region, deep down in our brain next to the hippocampus. The record of the word stores linguistic information such as the lexeme (that includes the lemma as well as possible markers for morphemes) and a tag as to what phonemes can be matched to the lexeme. If we encountered the word in written form, then information on spelling also becomes part of the record. Non-linguistic information, which may include emotional association, is transmitted by the senses when the word is encountered and rehearsed and, once recorded, also becomes part of the record. The non-mesial region itself is like an index of all those records of words.
3. Retrieval: The record of the word is called up from the non-mesial region. The lexeme and the tag are brought to Broca's area. The likelihood of activation depends on how the record of the word was created when the word was first encountered and processed. Phonemes are called up from Wernicke's area. Phonemes and lexemes are rehearsed subvocally in the phonological loop. Several lexemes are called up at once (L1 and L2 lexemes can be brought up simultaneously). The tag helps to discriminate the lexeme from other lexemes, as it has information regarding what phonemes can be matched to the lexeme. At the same time, the non-linguistic information

of the record of the word is reviewed. If necessary, the hippocampus is consulted to get information on how the record was created. The hippocampus is linked to the amygdala to access emotions. In a different part of Broca's area, morphemes are processed and the word is encoded for speech production. Linguistic information between lexemes, phonemes, and morphemes, as well as non-linguistic information, are exchanged until the word is assembled.

A Record of a Word

In the following section, we focus on processing phonemes and lexemes. We will deal with morphemes later, as they are processed at a later stage, although it is important to note that they feed information back to the lexeme and phonemes and vice versa. In general, phonemes and the lexeme of a word need to be processed before they decay. Working memory functions to prolong the processing time so that the brain has the capacity to temporarily store some phonemes at the same time as other phonemes are rehearsed (Baddeley, 2007). This allows the language faculties more time to identify all of the phonemes of a word in order to match them to a lexeme. If the matching process is successful, a record of the word is created. The record can be temporary or permanent depending on the strength of the linguistic and non-linguistic information recorded. Each time our brain rehearses a word, its record is invigorated. Therefore, this process of rehearsal increases the likelihood that the word will be remembered. A strong record can be called up months and years after it has been created. This is what we know as long-term memory. If a word cannot be called up, the record was either initially too weak, or not maintained over time, as even a strong record requires maintenance. A weak record might be called up shortly after it was created but then dissipates. Therefore, key elements in word processing are rehearsal, repetition, and maintenance. With regard to repetition, spacing information in intervals is beneficial in order to complete a rehearsal process before the next one starts. We will discuss this in more detail in Chapter 7, "Spacing."

Several areas in the brain are involved when processing a word. In particular:

- Executive control (location: dorsolateral prefrontal region – responsible for directing, dividing, and switching attention)
- Phonological loop (two locations: left prefrontal cortex – responsible for rehearsal; and left side of the parietal lobe – responsible for temporary storage)
- Broca's area (location: left prefrontal cortex – responsible for production (some overlap with loop)

- Wernicke's area (location: left side temporal lobe – responsible for comprehension)
- Hippocampus (location: mesial temporal lobe deep down in the brain – responsible for creating a record of a word)
- Amygdala (location: mesial temporal lobe deep down in the brain – responsible for processing emotions)
- Enthornial and perirhinal cortices (location: mesial temporal lobe [left and right connecting several brain regions] – responsible for transmitting information from the senses)
- Non-mesial area (location: non-mesial temporal lobe – responsible for storing the record of a word)
- Auditory motor cortex (location: temporal lobe – responsible for processing sounds by frequency)
- Primary motor cortex (location: posterior frontal lobe – responsible for [among other things] coordinating our physical ability to speak such as lips and jaw).

In order to successfully process a new word, the brain's neurons fire simultaneously, the areas are activated and converge, and so transmit the necessary information (Singer, 2006; Tranel and Damasio, 2002). In addition, some of the areas form circuits to exchange information more quickly (Garagnani, Wennekers, and Pulvermüller, 2006; Pulvermüller, 1996). We need to note that these areas and circuits that allow us to acquire words are developed and refined over time.

The processing of a word takes place in several phases, and the phases overlap. As mentioned, in the first phase, the word needs to be attended to (Schmidt, 1995, 2001). Attention requires much energy and is linked to executive control. To be able to control attention means to be able to direct attention to an incoming word, to divide attention if there are several words incoming, and to switch attention if a new word that is particularly interesting is incoming (Baddeley, 2007). This is a very complex process involving several areas in the frontal lobe; therefore we have to decide which word we pay attention to when we first hear it and which one we ignore because we deem it to be not relevant. Our attentional resources are limited (Robinson, 2003; Skehan, 2009a). If not relevant, there is no need to start the process, because we can use the necessary energy for other words. In the second phase, the language faculties such as those of the phonological loop and Wernicke's area (for recall: Broca's area), as well as the memory faculties such as the hippocampus, are activated. The hippocampus, a protected region deep down in the brain, creates a record of the information that has been processed, and is connected by neuroanatomical circuits to the amygdala as well as to the enthornial and perirhinal cortices that also sit deep down in the brain (Tranel and Demasio, 2002). The hippocampus, amygdala, and the two cortices are part of the temporal lobe and form an area called the mesial temporal lobe. They are represented on the left and right side of the brain.

The amygdala plays a key role in the processing of emotions, which in turn play a role when recording information (Tranel and Damasio, 2002). If a word is tagged by the amygdala and consequently fast-tracked, its lexeme and phonemes are processed with heightened activation. The amygdala achieves this through its many connections not only to the enthornial and perirhinal cortices that transmit sensory information, but also to the basal forebrain (Amaral et al., 1992), which is connected to Broca's area. This heightened activation stimulates the memory trace. A memory trace is the duration of time it takes a lexeme and the phonemes of a word to be processed before they decay. Most words decay in half a second, but the trace can be prolonged to last up to two seconds. With more stimulation, the likelihood of the lexeme to be matched to the phonemes increases. This happens with emotional words. For example, the probability of processing a word like "hot" is higher compared to a word like "hat," even though they are only differentiated by one letter. "Hot" has many potential emotional associations, like "hot weather," "hot car," or "hot coffee." The enthornial and perirhinal cortices connect the hippocampus so it can receive sensory information from other brain regions; for example, visual, auditory, or olfactory information (Gluck and Myers, 2001). Sensory information is processed in different brain regions: the visual cortex is part of the occipital lobe at the back of the brain; the auditory cortex connects ear to ear as part of the temporal lobe; and the olfactory bulb, which sits under the frontal lobe close to the nose, processes smell. All these cortices are represented on the left and right side of the brain. In summary, the procedure of creating a record is not limited only to the left side of the brain where the phonological loop, Wernicke's, and Broca's area are located, but rather the convergence of activity across many regions highlights the brain's interconnectivity as it processes words.

In order to retrieve a word to speak it, these brain areas are activated again. The retrieval of a word can be triggered by emotions or by the executive control, or both. If a word cannot be recalled right away, the amygdala can be activated by stimulating the senses, which may in turn assist memory. This works well with words that are attached to an emotional situation or event. For example, imagine you burned your tongue the first time you drank a coffee in Germany. You may then more easily recall the German word for "hot" ["heiß"]. The executive control can also signal that a particular word is needed in order to respond to the other person in a conversation. In order to process a word for speaking, the word is prepared by Broca's area in consultation with Wernicke's area, the two being connected with subcortical fibers. The record of the word is called up into the loop of Broca's area from the non-mesial region. The record includes lexemes (with their lemmas and morphological markers) and a tag that indicates which phonemes can be matched to the lexeme. Lexemes and phonemes are rehearsed until the word is processed fully. If needed, the hippocampus is contacted. The process of generating a word for speech production is self-monitored. Monitoring takes place when the lexeme is matched to the phonemes. It is not quite clear where exactly that happens in the brain, but in general it involves the left side of the temporal lobe (Indefrey and Levelt, 2004). The temporal lobe houses the auditory cortex, as one function of monitoring is to hear, subvocally, the pronunciation of the word. At a slightly later stage morphemes are attached to the lexeme. This also occurs in Broca's area. Morphemes feed information back to lexemes and phonemes until the correct morpheme is found. If it is not found, there are two scenarios. One, the word is produced without a or with an incorrect morpheme which will result in a speech error; and two, the process of calling up a word will start all over again.

Another role of the primary auditory cortex, as well as the primary motor cortex, is to identify the prosody (stress, rhythm, and intonation) of the word and to train the vocal cords and the tongue to reproduce those sounds. Some linguists argue that prosodic features are also part of the record that is created, which would indicate that the process of new word acquisition is highly individualized, as every speaker hears and pronounces a new word with a slight, nuanced difference (Port, 2007).

Where is a word actually stored? The answer used to be that the record of the word is stored in the hippocampus, but that no longer seems to be true. Although the hippocampus does play a key role in how the brain processes a new word and creates a record, newer studies have shown that the permanent storage area is likely in the neocortices adjacent to the hippocampus (O'Connor, Butters, and Miliotis, 1992; Tranel, Damasio, and Damasio, 2000; Tranel and Damasio, 2002). These neocortices are found in the non-mesial temporal region of the temporal lobe. We will go into more detail later in the chapter.

For almost all right-handed, and most left-handed, people, there are four scenarios for how a word travels through the brain.

1a A new word is recorded

Imagine you are back at the airport drinking the very strong and very hot and very small coffee. You think about that word: "der Kaffee." What needs to happen in the brain so that you will be able to recall that word at any time in the future? First, the words "der Kaffee" needs to get your attention. If it does, an executive control function in the frontal lobe directs attention to the word. This happens in the upper part of the frontal lobe called the dorsolateral prefrontal region. The word has your attention because this coffee is different than your usual experience of coffee. The word is then rehearsed in the phonological loop (see Figure 3 for the overall process of rehearsal to storage).

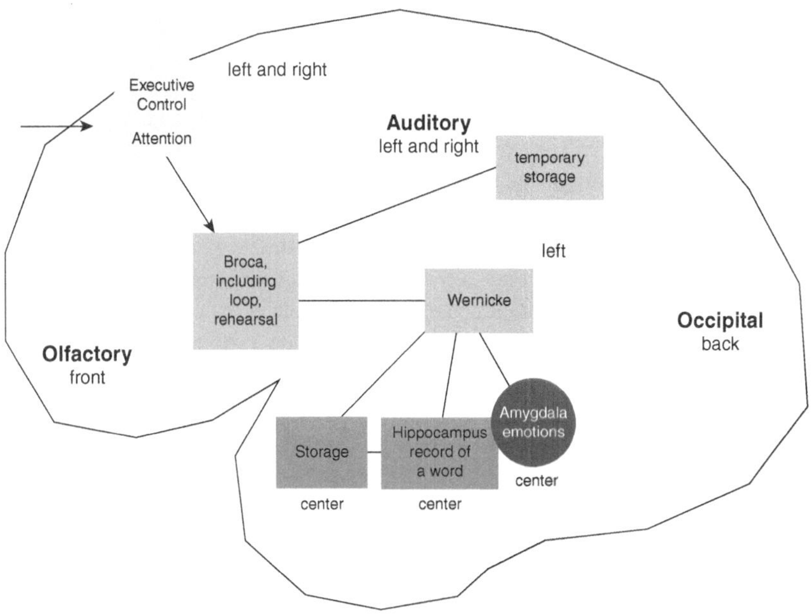

Figure 3. Rehearsal to Storage.

The loop has two subsystems: the rehearsal (part of Broca's area in the left prefrontal cortex), which recites the phonemes until they are identified; and the temporary storage (left side of the parietal lobe), where the phonemes are temporarily stored if they cannot be identified immediately. In order to identify them, Wernickes's area (located in the left temporal lobe and connected to Broca's area by subcortical fibers) is contacted, as that is where the repertoire of known phonemes is stored. The incoming phonemes are compared to those already in the repertoire. In order to compare and match the German phonemes to the ones you know, the loop will work together with Wernicke's area to rehearse English phonemes (if English is your first language) as well as German phonemes (if you know some German already). The rehearsal of "Kaffee" eventually forms connections among the phonemes. Identification takes place in the loop because all the phonemes of the incoming word must first be recognized before they can be processed. Once identified, the phonemes are matched to a lexeme. This takes place in Wernicke's area, which constantly exchanges information with the phonological loop. Furthermore, Wernicke's area contacts the non-mesial region, where the index of records of words that are already known are stored, to see if the new word matches a lexeme that is already known, in this case the lexeme of "coffee." Finding the lexeme, it is looking for a lemma that is linked to a concept. A lemma is part of a lexeme. Obviously, the concept of "Kaffee" is a bit different than the concept of "coffee," but there is still a similarity. Thus, the experience of drinking a "Kaffee" helps to trigger the concept.

In addition to matching the phonemes to the lexeme, Wernicke's area identifies the graphemes (in case you see the word "Kaffee" spelled out; for example, on the board behind the counter) and morphemes (if the word has any; for example, distinguishing singular and plural forms). If the phonemes and lexeme (and graphemes, if necessary) are matched, the word "Kaffee" travels to the mesial region, which is deep down at the base of the brain. The mesial region contains several components, including the hippocampus, the amygdala, and the enthornial and perirhinal cortices. The cortices feed information from the senses, such as images from the occipital lobe, sounds from the auditory cortex, or smells from the olfactory bulb, to the hippocampus, to aid the hippocampus to create a record of the word. The smell and texture of "Kaffee" might be recorded, in addition to an image of the café and music that was playing in the background. The record is then moved to the non-mesial region of the brain, near the mesial region, where it is stored.

1b An emotional word is recorded

Now you also want to remember the word "heiß," which means "hot." In general, the process is similar to the process with which you remembered "Kaffee." However, the variation here concerns the role played by the amygdala, important in emotional processes. When you take a sip of the coffee, your lips and tongue can feel that it is hot. This arouses the senses and alerts the amygdala, which heightens the processing of "heiß." In turn, the amygdala alerts the executive control and this attention results in further activation in the brain. The loop and Wernicke's area start processing and soon "heiß" is traveling to the mesial region, so the hippocampus can create a record of the word with the help of the senses via the enthornial and perirhinal cortices. All this interaction bolsters the link between the mesial region and the loop. First, the amygdala heightens the word to be rehearsed; second, the word is processed via Wernicke's area to the hippocampus. Third, the word is moved for storage to the non-mesial region, and here there is another difference to the word "Kaffee." In addition to storing the verbal information, you can be certain that the sensation of burning-hot liquid is also stored because of its strong emotional activation. If you actually happen to burn your tongue, this is even better – because, although the sensation is painful, the heightened activation in your brain makes it more likely that you will remember the new word.

2a A word is called up

Imagine you are staying in Germany for a few days. After that first experience with the "Kaffee," you switch to other drinks, such as a cappuccino. But now you crave a coffee. In order to get one, you need to remember the word "Kaffee." What happens in the brain when we want to call up a word from memory? First, there is the need to remember the word. The executive control area in the dorsolateral prefrontal region recognizes that need, so it calls up the word from the non-mesial region, where the record was stored after it was created by the hippocampus in the mesial region (see Figure 4 for the overall process of recalling a word from storage). Actually, the records of several words are called forward by the executive control. Each record includes the lexeme (with its lemma and morphological marker) and a tag that indicates the combination of the phonemes to the particular lexeme, information on spelling (if available), as well as non-linguistic information transmitted by the senses. At the same time, phonemes are called up from Wernicke's area. Phonemes and lexemes are rehearsed subvocally in the phonological loop. Rehearsal takes place in the subsystem of the loop that is in the left prefrontal cortex, which is part of Broca's area. Phonemes might be temporarily stored in the other subsystem of the loop in the left side of the parietal lobe that, if necessary, can prolong the time needed to assemble the word. The lexemes of the words called up simultaneously will be those similar in meaning to the desired word; that is, those that express similar concepts via the lemma as part of the lexeme, such as "Kaffee," "Espresso," "Tee." Also, lexemes associated with the word you are looking for can be called up, such as "Zucker" or 'Milch." All of these can be L1 and L2 lexemes. In addition, phonemes with similar sounds will also be called forward (such as [a] or [æ] for "a," or [e:] or [ɪ] for "ee"). They will need to be rehearsed by the loop in order to discriminate between them. The tag helps to identify the phonemes that can be matched to the lexeme. Finally, a particular combination (in this case, [a] and [e:] along with [K] and [f], matching "Kaffee" [Kafe:]) receives more activation than others and is selected. If necessary, Broca's area might also exchange information with the hippocampus. The record of a word includes information transmitted by the senses such as audio, images, or other sensual information, but if the desired word cannot be immediately identified, the hippocampus can help by reviewing how the record was created. In this case, non-linguistic information recorded alongside linguistic information can trigger the memory, in particular emotions. The smell and texture of "Kaffee" might also be recalled, the look of the coffee place, the music that was playing in the background. Broca's area processes the word further by assigning bound or system morphemes, together with where the word is placed in a sentence. For example, if you want to order two coffees in English, you need the plural form of coffee marked by the morpheme "-s." The German language has many more morphemes, because there are many ways for nouns to form the plural. In the case of "Kaffee," though, it is a null-morpheme because two coffees is "zwei Kaffee" with no change to the noun. Eventually, Broca's area has to come up with a pre-speech plan. In order to

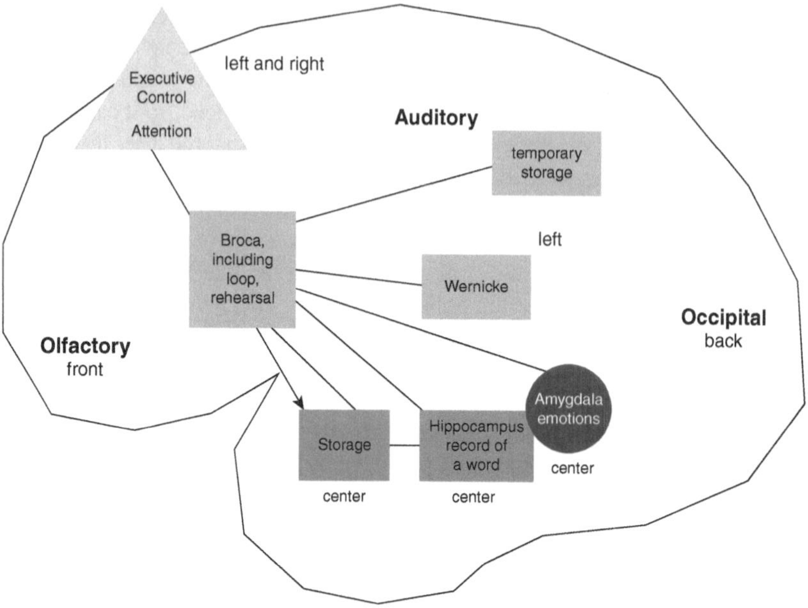

Figure 4. Recalling from Storage.

ensure the word is comprehensible and pronounceable, Wernicke's area and the auditory cortex review the plan before the word is spoken. If so, you say "Kaffee" and get what you want – even if this coffee is smaller and stronger than the one you first had in mind.

2b An emotional word is recalled

Now you also want to say the word "heiß," perhaps in connection with the words "nicht" and "so" in order to avoid burning your tongue again. In this case, "Nicht so heiß, bitte" means, "Not so hot, please." When we compare the word "Kaffee" to the word "heiß," we find differences in the recall process, as "heiß" was recorded with heightened activation and "Kaffee" may not have been. First, in addition to the executive control from the dorsolateral prefrontal region that calls up the record of the word, the amygdala, a primary player in emotion processes, will also become involved. This will activate the senses that were active when the record of the word was created. The amygdala is located in the mesial region, very close to the non-mesial region where the record is stored. This proximity means that communication is loud and clear between the mesial and non-mesial regions. In the non-mesial region, the sensory properties of "heiß" were stored alongside the verbal information of "heiß," which created a strong record. Consequently, our brain should be able to quickly recall and evaluate such a strong record. In the loop, the word is rehearsed and prepared for speech production by Broca's area. The hippocampus can be activated for additional sensory information but this may prove unnecessary since the activation of "heiß" was already so vivid. The word is monitored and if everything is approved, it is spoken.

Creating the record of a word, we must keep in mind that more information goes through the enthornial and perirhinal cortices than is recorded in the hippocampus. We cannot record everything. So how do we increase the likelihood that a word we want to process will in fact be recorded? The answer is that the word needs our attention, meaning that we must first determine if it is important. If we can, we should record not just linguistic, but non-linguistic, information that comes with the word, thereby activating our senses. Also, if we encounter the word several times over a longer time period we will give the loop the opportunity to rehearse it repeatedly. As a method, we can repeat words if there is a pause in between each repetition to ensure that the loop stopped processing the first rehearsal. If there is no pause, it will function as one long rehearsal, which is not as efficient. We return to this issue in Chapter 7, "Spacing."

Another question asks how long a word is recorded for. In general, the hippocampus can secure and retain memories for different durations. It can range from weeks to years to many years. However, most of the information stored in the non-mesial region will start to fade if it is not attended to every so often. How long the record will last before it fades will depend on how robust the record was when first created. When we recall, rehearse, and attend to the word, the record is renewed and the synapse is maintained. We will learn more about on maintenance in Chapter 3, "Synaptic Connections."

Some evidence on the workings of the phonological loop comes from studies with children who have an SLI. In such cases, the impairment can be isolated and the workings of the loop, Broca's, and Wernicke's areas, as well as the hippocampus, can be analyzed. These children have normal cognitive functioning and normal scores of general intelligence, which helps to isolate the effect of a language impairment on the ability to process new words. SLI is often genetic in nature. It can have many forms. Children might not be able to pronounce words correctly, to process words, to correctly attach grammatical forms to words, or to correctly order words in a sentence. In general, it has been suggested that children who have these SLI show a rapid decay of the memory trace, which causes insufficient processing because there is not enough time to rehearse the phonemes and match them onto a lexeme (Bishop, Adams, and Norbury, 2004). The good news is that if these impairments are detected early, in particular before the age of three, they can be treated, and over half of the children who suffer from SLI will have normal speech by the time they are six to eight years old. Further conclusions on this topic can be drawn from a 1990 study that compared children with an SLI to children with no language impairments (Gathercole and Baddeley, 1990). On standardized tests, the children with SLI had vocabulary and reading scores below average but had nonverbal intelligence scores in a normal range. The average age of participants was 8 years and 6 months, but their scores were comparable to children aged 6 years and 6 months to 7 years with no impairment. All the children did the same non-word repetition test that was used in a 1989 experiment by the same researchers. They repeated non-words of one, two, three, and four syllables. Interestingly, the children performed well on the one- and two-syllable non-words but their scores were very low on the three- and four-syllable non-words. The same test was carried out with two other groups of children, both with normal vocabulary and reading scores. One group consisted of children of the same age (8 years and 6 months) and the other of a younger age, in order to reflect the scores of the children with SLI (6 years and 6 months to 7 years). The scores of both of those groups on the non-word repetition test were high regardless of the number of syllables. By comparing the scores with two controls – same age, as well as younger children – it is clear that the difficulty of repeating non-words negatively impacts the vocabulary and reading skills and not vice versa. If low vocabulary knowledge impacted the ability to repeat non-words, the younger group (age 6 years and 6 months) would have had low non-word repetition scores. Particularly evident in this study are the problems children had with non-words of three or four syllables. In the loop, there is limited time to rehearse phonemes. If phonemes cannot be identified, they can be provisionally parked in the temporary storage of the loop. Therefore, it can be concluded that these children had impairment to the function of the storage area. This presented evidence for the separation of the loop into two subsystems (rehearsal vs. temporary storage), located in two different areas of the brain.

Why are we sometimes unable to recall a word we have already learned? There can be several reasons. One is that the record was never very strong, making the discrimination process difficult. We were able to recall it before because at that time other words (usually we speak in sentences) facilitated our recollection of the desired word in context. Another reason could be that too much time has passed since the desired word was last recalled. For example, perhaps it has been too many years since you were last in Germany and ordered a "Kaffee." In such cases, it is difficult for the central executive to activate the non-mesial region.

Sometimes, however, the record of the word is too strong. This can happen with emotional words. The lexeme that expresses a concept via the lemma was recorded with such strength that it does not accept any variation of the concept. Therefore, we sometimes have difficulties expressing what we feel in words. This is strictly linguistically speaking, as naturally there can be many other reasons why we sometimes cannot find the right word. This begs the question as to whether or not emotional words are easier to learn than non-emotional words. When we encounter an emotional word for the first time in another language, it is fast-tracked due to the corresponding heightened activation in the brain. An emotional word is also recalled more swiftly, as it has a strong record that makes the discrimination process easy. But what if the concept only exists in one language but not the other? For example, the German word "Angst" is a mix of "anxiety" and "fear." It has been imported into the English language, as neither English word expresses the concept of "Angst." Does the fast processing and swift recalling of the record of an emotional word outweigh the issue with its concept? Do we recall emotional words with greater success than other words in a second language? We will learn about concepts tied to emotions in Chapter 6, "The Bilingual Lexicon and Speaker," and about processing emotional words in another language in Chapter 8, "Word Analysis."

Storage of Words

Two questions need to be addressed with regard to the storage of words in our brain. What is stored? Where is it stored?

What is stored is the record of the word. The record is made of linguistic and non-linguistic information. The non-linguistic part of the record includes information on images, audio, smell, taste or touch, and emotions. The linguistic information contains the lexeme and a tag to the phonemes of the word. The lexeme itself consists of the lemma that is linked to a concept, as well as a morphological marker that is linked to a morpheme. The record also includes information on graphemes. The interesting thing is that phonemes, morphemes, and graphemes as such are not part of the record. There are only tags to link them to the record. Therefore, the record of a word only contains the bare essentials. The question is, of course, why?

The answer is a matter of efficiency. There are more than 100,000 words in most languages. That means there are more than 100,000 lexemes. However, the number of phonemes, graphemes, and morphemes is quite limited in any language. For example, English has between 36 and 48 phonemes and 26 graphemes, depending on the type of English spoken (for example, British English, American English, Australian English), whereas standard German has 45 phonemes and 30 graphemes. Therefore, it is more efficient for the brain to assemble the necessary parts of a word, rather than to process the word as a whole. It can be argued that to store a word as a whole takes up the same space as it does to store the lexeme of a word. For 100,000 words, there are also 100,000 lexemes. However, it is not so much a matter of space but of processing speed. Imagine every word with its lexeme and phonemes is stored in a one-to-one fixed state. To recall a word, one would have to go through each state until the correct one emerges. Of course, a hierarchy could be established in order to group words by theme when they are stored; for example, the word "coffee" could be stored under a category like "food and drinks." The problem is that, when trying to recall the word "coffee," we activate how the word was recorded. The situation in which the word was first encountered and all subsequent experiences influence the recall of the word. A hierarchy would therefore not be very helpful because our brains remember all the situational information. Try, for example, to remember a song by Bruce Springsteen. What is the best way to find it? Should you scan every song in an online library that has 100,000 songs in it? Or should you look it up under the category of "Rock"? Did you file it under "Rock"? Or did you file it under "Alternative"? How about "Soundtrack"? Or "1980s"? "Favorite Albums"? It might be faster to remember the melody (phonemes) and some of the meaning (lexemes), and then put two and two together.

There is always the possibility that the word will be assembled incorrectly. Phonemes are combined into syllables and therefore there are many possible combinations. Although phonological rules dictate the sequences of phonemes that are allowed and not allowed, we sometimes make errors and assign phonemes to a lexeme that does not match. When this happens, what comes out is something slightly incomprehensible. For example, "A cfofee with two pieces of sugar, please!" Interestingly, these errors prove that the stored linguistic record of the word consists of the lexeme and a tag indicating possible combinations of this lexeme to phonemes. If the phonemes were stored with the record, then such types of errors would not happen. We will learn more about errors in Chapter 4, "Cognitive Load."

There is another distinct advantage to the brain's practice of storing the record of a word that helps to match lexemes and phonemes. If the speaker acquires another language, s/he can draw on existing resources. A lexeme includes a lemma and a morphological marker. The lemma ties the lexeme to a concept and can be shared across languages. In the initial stages, much of what we learn in another language is based on the process of transfer from L1 to L2 lemmas. If each word were stored as a fixed unit, we would have to go through a new set of 100,000 words to find the desired word in the new language. On the other hand, calling up the record allows the speaker to use the L1 lexeme to quickly find the L2 lexeme. Nevertheless, once the lexeme has been identified, a morpheme must still be added via the morphological marker.

Neuroscientists and others have debated the question of where exactly the brain stores words (Milner, Squire, and Kandel, 1998). Initially, it was thought that the hippocampus both created and stored the record of a word. However, subsequent studies showed that damage to the hippocampus did not have a substantial impact on word recall. Does the brain have an alternate storage location for the record of a word, in addition to the well-protected hippocampus? It does. It can be argued that to have a separate storage location, such as the nearby and equally well-protected non-mesial region, is inefficient. However, it can also be argued that having one region creating a record of the word (hippocampus) and another region storing the word (non-mesial region) provides a safeguard. If the hippocampus is damaged, it is difficult to create new records and thus learn new words. However, those words already learned can still be recalled. This is precisely what some studies have found.

One particularly well-studied case concerns the patient known as PV (Baddeley, Papagno, and Vallar, 1988; Basso et al., 1982; Vallar and Baddeley, 1984). PV suffered a stroke at the age of twenty-six to the left hemisphere of the brain. PV spoke Italian as a first language. During one version of the test, researchers presented PV with a visual list of words (in Italian), and, after a short pause of a few seconds, asked her to recall as many words as possible. In this case, PV was able to recall a substantial number of words. However, if researchers presented words to PV orally, she had difficulties. If PV had to learn new words, she could not. The test on new words provided even more specific information. First, researchers gave PV the first word in Italian followed by a second word with a similar meaning. As Italian was her first language, she knew both words. Next, researchers prompted PV with the first word, and then asked her to speak the second word. For example, using our example of "coffee," the first word would be "warm" and the second word "hot." PV was able to give the second word on most trials. In the next part of that study, researchers gave PV the first word in Italian and the second in Russian, a language she did not know and which has no resemblance to Italian in either phonology or morphology. PV was not able to give the word in Russian when prompted by the Italian word, in particular when the Italian word was presented orally and not visually. This showed that PV had suffered damage to Wernicke's area (speech comprehension), as well as the hippocampus, which made it difficult to process a new word. However, she could recall words, via the non-mesial region, that had been learned before the stroke occurred. These words had been recorded by the hippocampus when the hippocampus was intact. This supports the theory that the storage of words cannot occur in the hippocampus. Furthermore, PV's difficulties with words presented orally indicated damage to the phonological loop, most likely to the temporary storage but not to the rehearsal, as she was still able to utter words. Interestingly, suffering a stroke to the left hemisphere one could normally expect damage to Wernicke's area and the phonological loop, but not necessarily to the hippocampus.

Other research studied the effects of time on memory, and showed that older memories are longer-lasting (Milner, Squire, and Kandel, 1998). This was later supported by Tranel, Damasio, and Damasio (2000).

Tranel and his colleagues carried out a study with participants who had suffered ischemic anoxia, a type of stroke to the brain. The ischemic anoxia attack disrupts the flow of blood to the brain, which means the brain consequently does not receive enough oxygen. If the attack goes on for several minutes, part of the brain shuts down and usually does not recover. The brain tissue in the affected region dies. Tranel et al. found that damage to the hippocampus alone had less of an impact than damage to the hippocampus and the entorhinal cortex, which thereby underscores the function of the cortex to transmit information from other brain regions to the hippocampus in order to assist in the creation of a word record. This suggests evidence for the theory that creating a record in the mesial region and storing the information of that record in the non-mesial region has the advantage of providing a safeguard. We can also consider the opposite scenario: not the mesial, but the non-mesial, region is damaged. If the non-mesial region is damaged, words that have been learned, and old memories in general, cannot be recalled. However, new memories can be formed and recorded, but there is the difficulty of storing them for longer periods of time.

As with the workings of the phonological loop, the precise function of the hippocampus has been analyzed with the help of research on patients with brain damage. In the section on memory loss in this chapter, we will discuss in more detail studies that are very important to our understanding of how words are processed. The development of current neuroimaging technology has been instrumental to new research; however, as some researchers point out (Müller and Knight, 2006), neuroimaging is not an exact science and scans or measures of blood flow can be misinterpreted. It is therefore important to continue in-person studies that ask patients with brain damage or brain illness to engage with word tasks or recall of lists of words in the presence of a researcher.

With regard to the technology available today, the following four methods are best able to analyze what happens where in the brain when words are processed:

- PET (positron emission tomography)
- fMRI (functional magnetic resonance imaging)
- MEG (magnetoencephalography)
- EEG (electroencephalography).

The above technologies monitor the brain at the same time as the patient performs a set task. In detail, PET measures blood flow. The patient receives an injection of a natural chemical such as glucose, ammonia, or water, which is also tagged with a radioactive tracer in a colored dye. The tracer then travels inside the natural chemical through the bloodstream to areas in the body that most use the natural chemical, for example, glucose travels to areas of the body that use glucose for energy. With the use of a scanner, a radiologist can then monitor the route and destination of the radioactive tracer and interpret the results.

The fMRI technique creates a strong magnetic field to measure blood flow. An increased blood flow in a particular part of the brain indicates an increased activation in that area, as a brain area that is active needs more oxygen. The fMRI scan makes use of hemoglobin, an iron-rich protein found in red blood cells. The iron makes it detectable when a magnetic field is created. Using the fMRI technique, the magnetic field is constantly changed to detect the blood flow.

An alternative to fMRI is to measure magnetic mismatch negativity (MMN) with a technique called magnetoencephalography (MEG). In this approach, the naturally occurring magnetic fields of neural circuits are measured with a highly sensitive magnetometer device. A participant performs two different tasks while the magnetic field that occurs during the first task is compared to that of the second task.

EEG measures brain activity by mapping the electrical current in neurons. Electrodes are placed on the scalp of a patient and over time record the electrical current, creating a waveform that researchers can look at.

Technology has its limitations. In theory, we can measure which brain regions are activated when a participant performs a word task. However, measuring the level of activation – that is, how much of the activation is related to lexical processing and how much is general cognitive functioning – is difficult to distinguish. Another problem is that, depending on the technique, the spatial or temporal resolution is low. We know, for example, that Broca's area is activated when we speak. However, Broca's area itself is complex. Phonemes, lexemes, and morphemes interact with one another. The spatial resolution is usually not high enough to determine the details of this interaction. Further, the participant must be very still, so the scan will not be distorted. Therefore, many studies test comprehension by having a participant press a button when they recognize a word. For linguistic purposes, however, we want to know what happens during speech, specifically, lexical production. A common task used in neuroimaging studies is called the "n-back task." This is a task that consists of two rounds. In the first round, a series of letters or words is presented to the participant followed by a break. The words chosen are usually similar in length. They are also similar on how they rank on the frequency list. Most languages have a list of the most-used words, which are ranked from 1 to 1,500 or more. The study has to make sure that the words tested do not rank low on the frequency list (meaning that they are rarely used and therefore very likely new and unknown to the participant). After the break, in the second round, letters or words are presented again, some of which have also been presented in the first round. The participant has to indicate, by pressing a button, if s/he has already seen the letter or word in the first round. The task therefore focuses on comprehension only. This helps to localize the brain regions activated, but it does not reflect the entire process. To acquire a new word also means to be able to recall that word when needed. In order to analyze recall, studies use what is called a "free recall task." The first round is similar to the "n-back task," where words are presented in succession. In the second round, the participant is asked to recall as many words as possible. This task does indeed measure what is required from a language learner who needs to recall words of the L2. However, so many regions are simultaneously activated when the brain processes and recalls words that it is difficult to monitor and localize precisely what happens where and when.

In the case of PET, the biggest problem is temporal resolution, because the radioactive substance does not travel very fast. The region may in fact have been activated, but may not show activation by the time the radioactive substance arrives. An advantage of PET is that participants can carry out speech-related tasks during the test, although in order to minimize movement participants must say or read out loud single words at a time.

In fMRI scans, the magnetic field has to be constantly changed, and this also takes time. In addition, fMRI studies are problematic in that the participant must be perfectly still. That means the person cannot speak, because the movement of the jaw would distort the scan. Therefore, studies rely on measuring reaction times by pressing a button. However, spatial resolution using fMRI is higher than with any other neuroimaging technique.

The MEG technique avoids the problem of time, as it measures a naturally occurring magnetic field. Unfortunately, the naturally occurring magnetic field is weak and difficult to detect, and spatial resolution is low. As in PET studies, participants can speak single words when tested.

EEG is not as commonly used as PET, fMRI, or MEG, because all it does is create a waveform. Furthermore, there is a time delay: the point of measurement at the scalp is not where the activity occurs inside the brain. Therefore, the electric waveform might be influenced by other factors, such as the central executive directing, dividing, or switching attention. On the plus side, as with PET and MEG, participants can perform tasks where they actively produce words.

What is measured using these techniques when we speak or hear another language? The faculties involved in language processes and recall – the loop; Broca's and Wernicke's areas; the hippocampus, cortices, and sometimes the amygdala; the senses; the non-mesial region – are the same in first and second language acquisition. Studies attempt to measure whether there is more activation of those brain regions during the processes of L2 compared to L1; if these brain regions indeed process L2 and L1 in an identical fashion or if there are variations within the faculties; and whether the answer might depend on the learner's level of proficiency and the phase of development. However, whereas neuroimaging studies can help to determine which neuroanatomical circuits the brain uses when it processes words in L1 and L2, neuroimaging techniques cannot help us to analyze how phonemes and lexemes are selected, rehearsed, matched, and later encoded with morphemes. At least, not yet.

In summary, the processes of word acquisition and recall are complex operations that involve many brain regions at once. We must keep in mind that the application of neuroimaging technology is still limited, since results vary according to the type of task performed by the participant. We must also note that neuroimaging studies often use participants with different types of brain damage. Consequently, studies using PET or fMRI scans, or MEG, or that measure electrical activity (EEG), do not always reach the same conclusions. We must examine each study rigorously, and ask who was analyzed, what was analyzed, and how the analysis was performed. Despite these constraints, technology continues to improve, which allows us to learn more about the brain.

One of the first studies using PET on the processing of single words came from Petersen et al. (1989), published in the first volume of the *Journal of Cognitive Neuroscience*. Adult native speakers of English heard English nouns – for example, "cake." In one of the tasks, the speakers repeated out loud the noun they had just heard. In another task, they had to name a verb that they associated with the given noun – for example, "to bake." The scan showed that the radioactive substance lit up Broca's area, associated with speech production, in the left prefrontal cortex. One of the first studies on the phonological loop, using an improved fMRI technology, was carried out by Wagner et al. (1998). There were two trials. In the first trial, healthy participants were shown lists of words. In order to encourage their attention, participants were asked to indicate/label the words as either abstract or concrete. There was a twenty-minute break. In the second trial, the words were shown again and participants were asked to indicate, by the press of a button, which ones they had already previously seen. The fMRI measured brain activity in both trials, and results showed that in the second trial participants exhibited more activity in the prefrontal cortex of the left hemisphere (phonological loop: rehearsal), as well as in the parietal lobe of the left hemisphere (phonological loop: temporary storage), when they remembered words than when they did not remember.

A new, emerging technology to analyze the brain comes from a technique called neurophotonics, which uses photons (units of light) to measure brain processes at the cellular level. Much of that research is carried out at Laval University in Quebec, at University of California, Davies, as well as at Australian National University in Canberra, where high-resolution microscopes allow researchers to see transmissions between neurons. The use of light to provide a high-resolution image of the brain presents numerous technical challenges. Within the neurophotonics technique a number of approaches are tested, each set to improve the depth that the light can go into the brain and still provide quality spatial resolution, as well as to improve temporal resolution, even if delays factor in the range of milliseconds. The main use of this technique is to diagnose brain disorders, for example, by the measurement of cerebral blood flow to determine how exactly neural circuits function and form connections, as well as how they configure the motor outputs necessary to our body movements. At this time, the technique has not yet been used to analyze language processes. Although it remains to be seen if this technique will be helpful in understanding how neural circuits associated with the language faculties operate, studies using this technique are certainly something to look forward to.

Memory Loss

When we investigate the conditions under which words are acquired, we try to gain knowledge about processing words. We can learn much when this process is interrupted or not functioning, or both. Studies on memory loss can be divided into two subcategories:

1. injuries – for example, caused by a stroke or car accident
2. illnesses – for example, Down's syndrome (affecting children early on in life) or Alzheimer's (affecting adults later on in life).

Problems associated with injuries are usually localized to one specific area of the brain, which means that researchers can more easily study the direct impact to language faculties. However, problems associated with an illness are usually more difficult to research, because the illness may affect many brain functions. This makes it difficult to determine if the speech deficit is caused by a deficit to the language faculties (such as the phonological loop or to Wernicke's [comprehension] or Broca's [production] areas); to the memory faculties (the hippocampus); to the senses that feed information about a word to the hippocampus; or to the executive control that directs attention to an incoming word.

This is one of the reasons why research on dementia is so multifaceted, as there are many angles to consider. In initial diagnosis of brain dysfunction, we often speak of a mild cognitive impairment (MCI). Only about half of the people with MCI later develop a form of dementia. There are four forms: Alzheimer's, vascular dementia, prefrontal dementia, and Parkinson's disease.

At around 70 percent, Alzheimer's is the most common of all dementia forms. It starts in the hippocampus. Alzheimer's makes it very difficult, if not impossible, to form new memories and, in addition, existing memories are also destroyed. The neurochemistry of Alzheimer's has to do with a peptide called BAP (beta-amyloid peptide) and a protein called tau (Ittner et al., 2010). BAP assists with the metabolic cycle and is usually cleaned out of the system by the amyloid precursor protein (APP) that is regulated by the ApoE gene. However, if the gene does not function properly,

BAP will stay in the system and attached itself to a synapse. This will cause an overactivation that eventually destroys the synapse. Therefore, the brain can no longer transport desired signals. In addition, BAP interacts with tau, the protein that helps to transmit information from one neuron to another via phosphates. The interaction of BAP with tau is deadly, because it sets off a compounding virus-like chain reaction that causes tau to produce too many phosphates, which then attack and destroy the neuron itself. These abnormal chemical reactions can be hereditary; or related to lifestyle habits, such as low incidence of physical exercise or low social activity; or related to depression, burnout syndrome, vitamin deficiency; or reduced thyroid activity. When we focus on the ApoE gene in Alzheimer's, we must remember that every gene has two sides, a positive and a negative pole; therefore, it is possible for the ApoE gene to be present but for the subject not to get Alzheimer's if, on the positive/negative balance, one inherits all the poles which are not associated with Alzheimer's.

Finding a treatment is difficult, as there are many ways BAP and tau can interact. The interaction is complicated by the fact that BAP exists in varying lengths, and tau in different versions. Besides the hippocampus, the area most affected by Alzheimer's is the prefrontal cortex, where planning takes place. In healthy subjects this area directs attention to an incoming word. However, when Alzheimer's is present, the subject cannot process words, since the words are not directed toward the phonological loop. Finally, Alzheimer's also impacts Broca's and Wernicke's areas. When dealing with patients, it is important to know that Alzheimer's gradually impacts language – starting with memory, followed by planning, and finally speech.

It is also important to know that there are three other forms of dementia that are less severe with regard to how they impact language: vascular dementia, prefrontal dementia, and Parkinson's disease. Vascular dementia is caused by small strokes or cerebral hemorrhages, but, unlike Alzheimer's, usually only one of the three areas (hippocampus/prefrontal cortex/Broca's and Wernicke's areas) is affected. Prefrontal dementia is quite different. It starts at a younger age in the prefrontal lobe and mostly impacts the executive control and to some degree speech (word processes as well as articulation). Parkinson's disease is characterized by an underproduction of the neurotransmitter dopamine, which results in uncontrollable bodily shaking, as the signals to control body movements are not going through properly. Eventually, those with Parkinson's disease find it difficult to control the tongue, jaw, and other parts of the mouth and used for speech.

In order to prevent the MCI that can accompany aging from turning into a form of dementia, we must develop and practice good lifestyle habits. Regular physical activity, regular social contact, positive work-life balance, and a healthy diet (vitamins!) can make a difference.

Much of what we know about processing words comes from studies with patients who suffer from aphasia. Aphasia can be caused by either an illness or an injury. The most common causes are head trauma, stroke, and brain tumor or brain infections. There are several types of aphasia.

The best known is Broca's aphasia, caused by damage to Broca's area, which is responsible for speech production. This is a type of non-fluent aphasia, meaning that patients have difficulties uttering words, as they cannot be rehearsed properly. Spoken sentences sound like old-style telegrams: "I car raining hit wake up hospital." It is believed that the problem is that there is too little activation of lexemes and phonemes to be processed sufficiently. These phonemes and lexemes are selected because there are no alternatives, since, due to the low activation levels, the process that normally discriminates them from other phonemes and lexemes has become dysfunctional. If lexemes and phonemes are not processed fully, it is almost impossible to attach morphemes later. Therefore, speech sounds ungrammatical. It consists mostly of content words (nouns, verbs, adjectives) that have no morphemes (such as 3.P.Sg. Present Tense "-s"). Function words (prepositions, conjunctions, some adverbs) are mostly absent.

Another type is Wernicke's aphasia. Here we have the opposite problem: an overactivation of lexemes and phonemes results in incorrect combinations of phonemes and lexemes because the loop is overburdened as it tries to sort them. The language is fluent, but the meaning is distorted. It is associated with damage to Wernicke's (speech comprehension) area. Patients make lexical errors, for example, they substitute one word with another word that may not be correct in that context; and sublexical errors, for example, they leave out certain phonemes, and add or change other phonemes within a word. The speech has a jargon-like character that is often incomprehensible, such as, "I cat raiming sleep pospitll." Interestingly, many people with Wernicke's aphasia do not realize that their speech is distorted, because their comprehension and speech-monitoring capability are also distorted.

Other types of aphasia include the loss of auditory comprehension, that is, a person is unable to comprehend spoken words but is able to speak. Semantic aphasia presents the inability to recall names for objects or generally having difficulties finding a word. These types of aphasia do not occur as often as Broca's or Wernicke's aphasia and therefore have not been as extensively researched.

3 Synaptic Connections

Neurons and Synapses

Neurons are nerve cells that can transmit information. A neuron is like a relay station containing three parts: dendrites, a nucleus, and an axon. The nucleus contains the genetic code that predetermines whether the cell has the capacity to transmit information. A synapse is the point of contact between two neurons. Where the neurons do not meet, the gap or space between them is called a synaptic gap. Information comes in the form of an electrical signal. The electric signal, known as a nerve impulse, is passed from one neuron to another at the synapse. Sometimes the signal can be quickly transferred at the synapse of two adjacent neurons, but if not it can then be carried across the gap through a biochemical process with the help of neurotransmitters. In the process of neurotransmission, the neuron releases a chemical – the neurotransmitter – which drifts across the synaptic gap and transports the message from the axon of one neuron to the dendrites of another. The dendrites of the receiving neuron convert the chemical message back into an electronic nerve impulse that can then be read by the nucleus of the receiving neuron and passed on to the axon. This is how nerve impulses can travel between neurons. Through this process, each neuron can communicate with innumerable others and this facilitates the interconnectivity of our brain.

The biochemical reaction between two neurons can provide either a temporary or permanent bridge between the synaptic gap. If it is permanent, a new synapse, or bridge, is formed. Where these synapses can be built is predetermined by the genetic code. Whether or not they are built, however, is a matter of stimulation. Bridging the gap temporarily can be compared to the action of a boat that ferries the information across. Unfortunately, the boat only runs for a few minutes or, in some cases, for a few hours. The information has been transported but it cannot be recalled again at a later time. In order to recall information at a later time – for example, a word – a synapse must be created to form an actual bridge that facilitates permanent access.

Sometimes, an existing synapse can be modified. Every time we recall a word, the record of that word needs to be accessed. It is accessed via the synapse that was formed. The synapse has two functions: it stores the record of the word; and it connects two neurons and thereby provides a permanent access path to the record. What we know about a word, the form and meaning – and how we use it – can change. When a synapse adds or deletes information, it becomes modified. Every time we recall a word, the biochemical process required to call up the record reinforces the synapse that stores the record. This kind of maintenance is important to keep it intact. The synapse can be an eight-lane highway overpass, a rural covered trestle, a tree trunk over a wilderness creek bed. The strength of the synaptic bridge depends on the strength of the record of the word as it was created. Regardless of the type of bridge, any bridge, including an eight-lane overpass, can fall apart if the construction crew does not care for it. An eight-lane overpass created through the repeated recall of information over a long period of time will last longer than a wobbly tree thrown across a creek bed. For example, the words used by the commentator when a team scored the winning goal in the World Cup final, and that scene, including the commentary, which gets replayed every so often, will be easier to recall for any viewer. Other words from the commentary during the final might be forgotten within a few days.

There are several neurotransmitters that affect signal transmission in the brain, including serotonin, dopamine, acetylcholine, and glutamate. Serotonin and dopamine are particularly interesting, as they are associated with emotions that can be recorded when a word is processed via the amygdala and cortices. While serotonin is associated with happiness, dopamine is associated with pleasure. What is even more important is that dopamine flows through the brain region that regulates the reward system (the striatum). Thereby emotions are balanced with reason: when we do well we expect a reward. Acetylcholine is also linked to the reward system, and is also associated with arousal and attention.

In the case of memory formation, when the word we have just encountered is processed, a synapse in the region is modified or an additional synapse is created. Transmitted as an electrical signal through a series of biochemical processes, the information – linguistic (matching phonemes to a lexeme) and non-linguistic (senses, emotions) – is secured in that very synapse. It is there that the consolidation of a signal or several signals forms a memory. In a way, memory is nothing but a synapse that allows us to recall the information required, because it created permanent access. And yet, nothing is permanent when it comes to synapses. The focus of this book is on the learning and maintenance of new words, so they can be recalled months and even years after they are first acquired. The ability to successfully recall a word depends on the strength of the synapse created when the word was recorded, and that in turn depends on factors we will discuss in the following chapters. These factors are related to:

- word groups (length, similarity, and emotional connotation) and categories (content and function words) (see Chapter 8)
- spacing (see Chapter 7)
- the learning situation (see Chapters 8, 7, and 9).

When we speak of the connections made between two neurons in the form of a synapse and the permanent access it creates, we must further distinguish that particular path from the overall network of language and memory faculties in the brain. The overall network includes the phonological loop (rehearsal and temporary storage), Broca's area (speech production; also includes rehearsal of the loop), Wernicke's area (comprehension), the hippocampus (creating a record of a word), and the amygdala, as well as the enthornial and perirhinal cortices that transmit information from the senses to the amygdala. Neuroanatomical circuits connect these faculties. In this network of neuroanatomical circuits, the perisylvian cortex has a role of particular importance that has been studied by Pulvermüller and his team at the MRC Cognition and Brain Sciences Unit in Cambridge using computational modeling (Garagnani, Wennekers, and Pulvermüller, 2006; Pulvermüller, 1996). In their studies, Pulvermüller and his team mostly measure MMN using the MEG technique. They detected weak magnetic fields in the perisylvian cortex, which they then attributed to different circuits in the brain that spring into action in response to the type of words processed. In one study, the researchers presented adult native speakers of Finnish with Finnish words (Pulvermüller et al., 2006). The researchers presented the words in bits and pieces: first they showed a fragment of a word and gave the participant time to identify it by speaking the whole word. If the participant did not know the word, s/he was asked to remain silent, and the researchers presented another fragment of the same word. This went on until the participant could identify the word. The researchers measured in milliseconds the exact point when a word was identified and traced how activation spread through the brain. This allowed them to determine timing and location, that is, which brain areas were activated and when activation occurred. In general, a word is identified in less than half a second. Likewise, to recall and speak a word also takes about half a second, sometimes a bit longer. There are variations within the circuits; for example, emotional words can take a short cut to recall by being fast-tracked by the amygdala. Overall, it is helpful to distinguish between:

- the overall network of language and memory faculties
- the circuits within the network that are linked to word groups and categories
- the synaptic connections to recall the record of a word.

This language network is built and predetermined by the genetic code as we begin to process language early in life. Almost three decades ago, Jacobs (1988) argued that most of that network is built in the first six years of life. Other researchers have since confirmed this theory but also argue that the network is not refined until our mid-twenties, in particular when it comes to memory (Korte, 2009). We also have to keep in mind that the brain is adaptive, that is, it changes throughout life by responding to challenges. An interesting theory in this regard is that of "scaffolding" (Stemmer, 2010). It operates on the assumption that throughout life new neuroanatomical circuits can be developed. An interesting question is what happens when the circuit is broken, for example, by brain damage or an illness. Depending on the type of brain damage or illness, alternate circuits can be built or not built, which then become part of the network.

Converging Zones

Synapses can be created and modified at any point over a lifetime, but they can also fall apart at any given point in life. A neuron actually contacts about 1,000 other neurons to transmit a signal (Herculano-Houzel, 2009). However, only some neurons will pass on the signal containing the information of the word such as the identification of phonemes and the lexeme they match. Once that information reaches the hippocampus, a record of the word is created and stored in the non-mesial region. The information is stored in the synapse that allows the record of the word to then be recalled whenever needed. In order for this process to work, neurons need to be firing simultaneously (Singer, 2006). Tranel and Damasio (2002) suggest we think of these processes as converging zones. When the brain is stimulated, information travels in many directions and converges to bring all pieces of the puzzle together. It is kind of like a chemical soup that starts to heat up. If a word was recorded with heightened activation of the senses – for example, the word "heiß" [hot] – the soup heats up faster. The idea of converging zones fits well with that of neuronal language circuits.

A study that supports the idea of neurons firing simultaneously and synchronizing their efforts was carried out by Fell et al. (2001) with nine patients who had been diagnosed with temporal lobe epilepsy. Fell et al. used EEG to analyze word recall of these patients. EEG is commonly used with epilepsy patients to measure neuronal activity in the brain that triggers seizures, the most common symptom of epilepsy. The study was carried out in Germany with native speakers of German, all of whom had undergone surgery and who were on seizure-inhibiting medication at the time of the experiment. Since surgery, none of them had suffered a seizure. Surgery revealed that each patient's hippocampus had been affected by sclerosis – the most common type of damage associated with temporal lobe epilepsy – resulting in the loss of neurons. The subjects were asked to complete a word recall task, using four to eleven letters per word. The researchers showed the subjects a series of German nouns, presented on a computer, one by one, in blocks of twelve. After each block of twelve nouns, subjects were instructed to count backwards starting at a number between 99 and 81. The task of counting backwards is a commonly used distraction tool in word recall studies meant to stop the process of rehearsal in order to facilitate a new learning process with each new block. It has been shown that this type of repetition is very successful when learning words. Thus, after the distraction task, the next block started by presenting the same twelve words in the same order. All in all, twenty blocks were presented. Afterwards, subjects had to recall as many words as possible. The average score was 29.7 percent, which is quite low in comparison to that of healthy subjects. Fell et al. measured the activity in the hippocampus and the rhinal cortex. The rhinal cortex includes the enthornial and perirhinal cortices, which feed information from the senses to the hippocampus, where the record of a word is created. They found that the hippocampus and rhinal cortex synchronized their activity as measured by the electric signals when the subjects started to learn the words and desynchronized their activity when the subjects stopped learning the words. Fell et al. argue that this type of synchronization requires very accurate timing of neural discharges within a range of a few milliseconds and that this type of timing initializes memory formation.

According to Singer (2006), who carried out many experiments on this, the synchronization of neuron activity allows the neural circuit to spring into action like an ensemble following a beat. Singer measured the beat to be 25 milliseconds. The conductors of this ensemble are the interneurons, which contact a sensory neuron to start the process of signal transmission. Numerous neurons are active at the same time and belong to numerous ensembles. When a word is processed – either to create a record or to recall it – the neuron has two tasks. First it needs to find out if it belongs to that particular ensemble and, second, if it does belong, it must begin to synchronize. We can see now why one neuron contacts about 1,000 other neurons, because only some of them will respond and transmit that specific information. Interestingly enough, of all the neurons we have in our brain, more are involved when reviewing information, such as recalling a word, than when processing new information, such as recording a word. We can also see how factors such as prosody and coarticulation play a role when processing words. Coarticulation refers to the process during which the speaker pronounces one sound, even as the next sound begins, thereby creating an overlap. Vowels and consonants carry cues as to how to make the transition to the next sound. Prosody refers to stress, rhythm, and intonation, each of which modifies the sound waves. Aligning the waves, we reveal the importance of synchronization: to change one or two letters in a word is to change all of the waves.

Ensembles, waves, and synchronization remind us of music. Like musicians, the neurons have to find the beat and, moreover, the melody. Levitin

(2008) who researches music at McGill University in Canada argues that song reinforces the process of remembering words. One of the cognitive components of music is rearrangement, and that is also true for language. Rearrangement means to combine and recombine sounds, with endless possibilities. If the prosody and melody reinforce sound waves, the words of the song should be remembered easily. Levitin argues that synchronization starts in our brains the moment we were born: parents sing lullabies to their children long before the children are able to speak. Therefore, by the time the child's language capacity starts to develop further, the neurons in the children's brain have already had some training in how to synchronize language through music. In order to turn words into song, we must modify coarticulation and prosody, but that is not all. To create a song, a piece of music, we must not only align words but find a melody that consists of many sound waves to reinforce the other waves. We know that, when singing a song, the levels of the hormone oxytocin increase in our body. The hormone is associated with feelings of joy, empathy, anxiety, and trust. If an emotional word is sung, the effect is even greater, as if all the waves are in sync, because, in addition to the hormone oxytocin, high amounts of serotonin and dopamine are released. Consequently, the words of a song are easier to remember when sung to music, particularly in the case of an emotional song with emotional words.

The importance of prosody and coarticulation also highlights the need to practice pronunciation as we acquire another language. Singing some of the words we need to learn is a good idea, although this might only work if you can actually carry a tune. For those who cannot sing or do not want to sing, some studies have investigated whether playing background music, in particular classical music, positively influences the acquisition of new words (De Groot, 2006; Furnham and Bradley, 1997). Results, however, were inconclusive, as those studies showed that playing classical background music helped some learners but not others. Very likely this has to do with two factors. First, it depends whether the language learner happens to like classical music, as this will release feelings of joy and will activate the hormone oxytocin; and second, if the type of music aligns with the sound waves of the words you are learning, as some types of music might assist in that process better than others, although this remains to be tested.

Electric Signals and Bio-chemical Reactions

A neuron is a nerve cell that is specialized to transmit information. The information must bridge the synaptic gap between two neurons in order to continue. The signal the information carries is electrical in nature. In some cases it can almost instantaneously bridge the synaptic gap; in other cases, a chemical reaction involving neurotransmitters, proteins, enzymes, and hormones is set in motion in order to bridge the gap. The neurotransmitters serotonin, dopamine, acetylcholine, and glutamate are particularly important. Serotonin, dopamine, and acetylcholine function as chemical messengers that drift from the axon terminals of neurons across the synaptic gap in order to reach the receptor sites of other neurons. The role of glutamate is somewhat different, as it works as a mediator.

Among neurons, we have to further distinguish between interneurons (the initial phase: the electrical signal leads to the first chemical reaction by releasing a neurotransmitter), sensory neurons (the relay: the main biochemical processes), and motor neurons (the receptor: receiving the neurotransmitter and converting it back to an electrical signal).

The strength of the signal, as well as repetition of the same signal, can cause changes in the neurotransmitter system that will eventually lead to the formation of a synapse that attaches to another neuron to form a permanent bridge. Groundbreaking research in this area has been carried out by Kandel, who started his research in the 1950s and was one of the first neuroscientists to fully explain the biochemical processes of long-term memory (summarized in his 2006 book *In Search of Memory*, written after winning the Nobel prize in 2000). The brilliance of his approach was in its simplicity: instead of studying complex organisms, he chose to study a sea slug of the species *Aplysia*. About 90 percent of the genes we find in human nerve cells are also found in slugs. The principle of information transmission is the same as it is for humans. An electric signal leads to a chemical reaction that is converted back to an electrical signal. The chemical reaction happens in the synapse that connects two neurons and it is necessary to bridge the gap between the neurons so the signal can travel from one neuron to the other. So, by studying a sea slug, we can draw conclusions that are relevant for humans. The advantage of studying *Aplysia* rather than humans is that *Aplysia* has only 20,000 nerve cells compared to the 85 billion we have as humans. Consequently, with *Aplysia* it is easier to study the cells. Furthermore, most of *Aplysia*'s cells are rather large – in comparison to ours – so any change caused by a stimulus can be observed with the help of a microscope. One must of course use a very good microscope. *Aplysia* is about 12 in (30 cm) long, weighs several pounds (1 kg), and breathes with gills. Kandel studied *Aplysia*'s protective reflex. When *Aplysia* is touched at a certain part near the gills, called sipho, it withdraws the gills to protect them. Kandel and his colleague Kupfermann found they could modify the reflex (Kupfermann and Kandel, 1969). If the sipho is repeatedly touched, the reflex weakens, as *Aplysia* may begin to notice that there is no need for the reflex, since the touching causes no harm. If the touch is heightened by an electro-shock, the opposite happens: *Aplysia*'s reflex is stronger and continues to be stronger even if the next touch is light. A sign that *Aplysia* remembered.

In this case, it remembered the pain. Next, Kandel and his colleagues found out that the type of stimulus influenced the duration of *Aplysia*'s memory to either withdraw the gills or not. If the touching of the sipho was done repeatedly without interruptions, *Aplysia* reacted the same way for the duration of a day. If the touch was done repeatedly with interruptions, that is, with pauses in between, *Aplysia* remembered her reaction for up to four weeks. All that was left to do was to study the electrical and chemical processes in *Aplysia* triggering these types of reactions. Actually, that was the tricky part and it took decades of research to fully explain how signals are transported and manifested in neurons.

There are numerous publications on the functioning of neurotransmitters. Kandel (2006) describes a typical scenario. Any type of stimulus causes the neurotransmitter serotonin to be released. Serotonin functions as a messenger. It starts the transport of the signal via an interneuron that attaches to a sensory neuron. Actually, it does not really attach, but comes close enough to start a chemical reaction. A calcium channel in the sensory neuron opens and consequently calcium ions can stream into the sensory neuron, where they bind to the enzyme calmoduline. If four calcium ions bind to calmoduline, it becomes active and functions as a second messenger. Calmoduline adds phosphate to other enzymes and manufactures cAMP (cyclic adenosine monophosphate), which in turn catalyzes the activity of a protein via a kinase. The neuroscientist Krebs, who discovered this in the 1960s (DeLange et al., 1968; Krebs et al., 1966) and received a Nobel prize in 1992, called it protein kinase A or PKA, because it was the first recorded discovery where a kinase modified a protein. At this point, when the kinase is in progress, there are two possible scenarios: one that leads to temporary access, and another that leads to permanent access.

The process of temporary access is less complicated. The protein kinase A triggers the production of the neurotransmitter glutamate. Glutamate binds to a receptor of the motor neuron. The release of glutamate allows sodium to enter the motor neuron via an ion channel and to depolarize the dendrites. In order to understand this, we have to know that every neuron has axons that send signals and dendrites that receive them. Within the cell is what is called an action potential: an electrical charge that is kept neutral unless a signal is transmitted. The transmission is caused by biochemical processes, but at this point the electrical charge needs to be depolarized for the signal to enter. In a way, the actual transmission is electrical, although the process behind it is biochemical. If the cell membrane is depolarized, sodium can briefly enter the motor neuron through the cell membrane channel until calcium closes the channel again. It is the sodium that boosts the signal through the neuron and accomplishes the mission of opening the cell membrane channels. This can last from seconds to minutes, during which the cell has heightened sensitivity.

The calcium is equally important, because otherwise the signal – in the case of *Aplysia*, the reflex – will never stop.

The second possible scenario is permanent access. The initial process of opening a channel and manufacturing cAMP is the same as in temporary access. However, then the protein kinase A decides to wander into the cell nucleus, where it activates a gene that in turn produces a new protein that builds a new synapse. In order to do so, it needs the support of another kinase called MAP (mitogen-activated protein) kinase. The MAP kinase sees the protein kinase A go by, and decides to join in on the action. The protein kinase A then activates a regulator in the cell nucleus called CREB-1 (cAMP response element binding protein), whereas the MAP kinase deactivates a regulator called CREB-2. CREB has the capacity to activate a gene. This is important, because a gene has the ability to change the structure and function of a cell. The gene then starts to produce a new protein and the new protein either modifies an existing synapse or forms a new synapse. The new synapse provides an additional link to the motor neuron. Consequently, signals can be processed faster and more reliably. Memory is simply a modified or new synapse that provides access to stored information. The information can be recalled because a permanent path has been created. However, it should be noted that nothing is permanent. Both kinases – protein kinase A and MAP kinase – are needed in these processes. While protein kinase A activates a gene, MAP kinase deactivates another gene. The deactivation of that gene is necessary for the other gene to go to work. Otherwise, new synapses would be formed all the time.

In general the process works similarly with the neurotransmitters dopamine and acetylcholine, as they also open calcium channels when a signal is transmitted from one neuron to another, thereby allowing ions to enter the cell. For dopamine, there are two different types of receptors: D1-dopamine increases cAMP and D2-dopamine decreases it. This shows the important role that emotions play in memory processes, since the amount of cAMP will determine if the signal is temporary (with the help of sodium channels crossing to a motor neuron) or permanent (with the help of a gene building a synapse that attaches to a motor neuron).

The journey of a word from first encounter to storage is illustrated in Figure 5. The language faculties are highlighted in light gray, the memory faculties in medium gray, and the emotions in dark gray. The word "Kaffee" can be easily identified if English is your first language. The dotted lines indicate the rehearsal process that is in progress; the solid arrows, the rehearsal process that has been completed. Most words would have to be encountered several times, with pauses in between each encounter, in order to store them in the form of a synapse in long-term memory. The process illustrated here would have to be repeated several times.

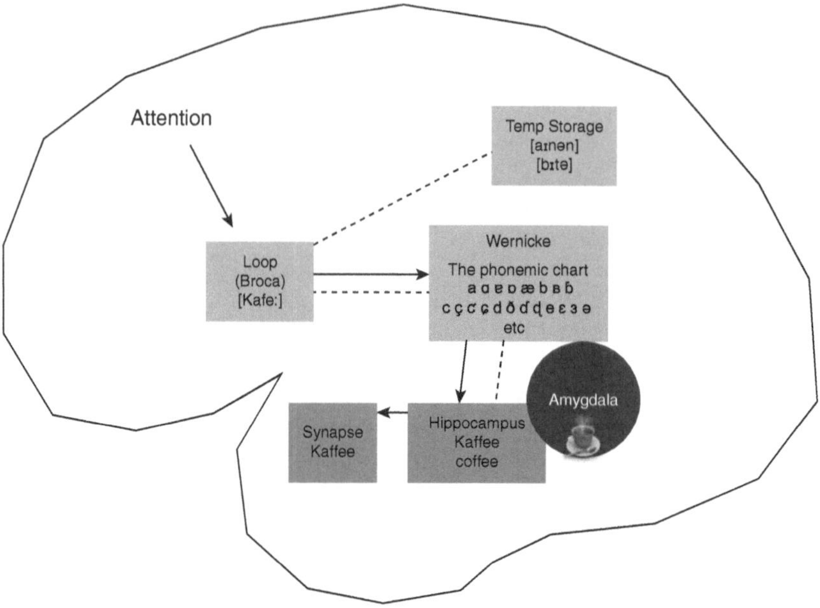

Figure 5. A Word's Journey through the Brain: First Encounter.

Recalling a word, we try to process the word we are looking for properly on the first attempt, which is illustrated in Figure 6.

How can we link temporary and permanent access to memory? The processes of working memory are temporary by nature: its function is to prolong a memory trace so there is more time to process it. However, the trace will vanish. The process is purely chemical and electrical, without a gene stimulating the formation of a synapse. Permanent access, on the other hand, means that a synapse allows us to recall information. We have to distinguish between short-term gains (recalling information minutes or days later) and long-term memory (recalling information weeks or month later). In short-term gains, the synaptic connection is fragile. After walking over a wobbly tree to get to the other side of a creek once or twice, it can collapse if no further construction is carried out. Recalling the word a few more times constructs a record of the word and it is then committed to long-term memory. This construction is that of a solid bridge one can walk over often.

The question then is, what is the threshold required to cause cAMP to drift into the cell nucleus? Kandel and his colleagues found out that one injection is not enough to start that process, but that several injections are required. If the number of repeated injections is five, cAMP will most likely start its journey into the nucleus. However, there is an exception. A single injection can also

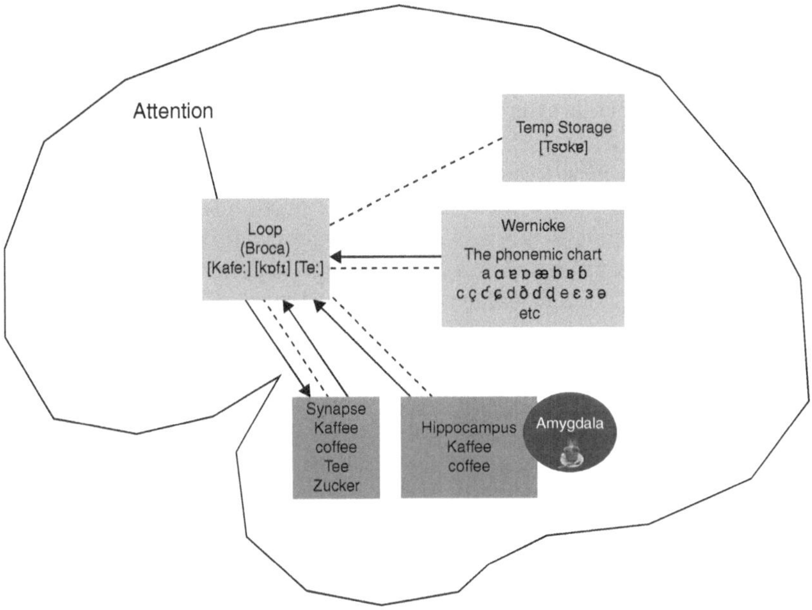

Figure 6. A Word's Journey through the Brain: Recall.

lead to the modification or formation of a synapse if the stimulation is very powerful. This implies that emotions can trigger such stimulation, as in a situation of high emotion a higher dose of serotonin will be released at once.

This is to say, to return to our coffee story, that if you learn the word "heiß" at the same time as you burn your tongue on a cup of coffee, at the airport in Frankfurt, on your first trip to Germany, you – in theory – will be able to recall that word quickly whenever you need it, as it was recorded with heightened activation. If you hear the same word "heiß" for the first time as it is spoken to you in a relevant sentence, such as, "Ist der Kaffee heiß genug?" (Is the coffee hot enough?), the activation is not as heightened. When you hear "heiß" in conjunction with an explanation that it means "hot," your memory will still call up an emotional association with that word, which might lead to the word's uptake to long-term memory. However, in the case of verbal communication vs. experiential learning, the uptake is not as fast or immediate as if you were to burn your tongue, because the burning sensation that triggers your emotions and senses, and thus leads to a more intense sensory experience, is absent. This does not mean, though, that in order to quickly learn new words in another language one must experience physical pain.

Something to know about serotonin is that it can be stimulated by estrogen. Women have high levels of estrogen and therefore seem to have a natural advantage over men when they process information, particularly if the information is emotional in nature. Future research on this topic could include a study that seeks to compare the rate of recall for men and women as they attempt to acquire new words that have an emotional connotation. We will discuss recall rates in more detail in Chapter 8, "Word Analysis."

Such scientific findings reveal information important to our understanding of how new words are processed in second language acquisition. If a word is only encountered once, it is unlikely that a synapse is formed that will then hold the record of that word. However, if the word is an emotional word or is tied to an emotional event processed with heightened activation, then the likelihood of synapse formation and the creation of a permanent record increase. Likewise, to repeat a word increases the odds that a new synapse will be formed or modified, which increases the strength of the word record. However, these processes also depend on the interval and time frame in which the word is repeated. It is unhelpful to repeat a word five times in a row, since the same biochemical reaction is in progress, which does not provide time for a new biochemical reaction to occur. When a word is repeated with pauses in between each new repetition, a new biochemical reaction takes place, and a synapse can eventually be formed which will store the record of the word in the non-mesial region. The questions, then, are those we asked in the Introduction:

- How often does a word need to be repeated?
  How does this rate of repetition relate to word groups when we distinguish between numbers of syllables (word length), similarity (in meaning [lexemes], pronunciation [phonemes], both [lexemes and phonemes]), and/or emotional connotations or situations?
- What type of repetition (interval) needs to be used?
  Which is of greater benefit to the creation of a synapse: a uniform interval where the same amount of time elapses between each repetition, or an expanded interval where the time lapsed from one repetition to the next increases? Or does it matter?
- What does the overall time frame look like?
  How often does a word need to be repeated? Should the same word be repeated within one learning session of seconds or minutes, or over multiple learning sessions over several days within a week or within a month? At what point in time can we assume that a synapse has been created to store the record of the word?

Chapter 7, "Spacing," attempts to answer the above questions in more detail. Notably, everyone's brain is different depending on the genetic code that predetermines the structures developed in each individual's brain. In addition to genetics, environment and upbringing also influence one's brain development, with particular consideration to how and if we learn a second language. Finally, brain structures change throughout life depending on the blood flow that carries oxygen and chemicals through the brain. We will return to that in Chapter 5, "First and Second Language Acquisition."

Neurogenesis and Synaptic Plasticity (Maintenance)

Many brain regions are involved in the processes of word acquisition and recall, which in turn require heightened attention and consequently much energy. When we acquire a word for the first time, brain activation levels are particularly high. In addition, because word encounter or recall contributes to the maintenance of a word record, the word also requires some form of cognitive attention with each time it is processed. In order to understand the factors required to maintain a word, we need to distinguish between two processes, which are based on the principle that our brain responds to change. These are called neurogenesis and synaptic plasticity. They evolve differently in our brain:

Neurogenesis (Formation of New Neurons)

Neurogenesis refers to the creation of new nerve cells. At birth, there are about 100 billion neurons. The number of neurons decreases as we age, although recently researchers have proved that the loss of neurons is not as dramatic as first thought. An adult brain has about 85 billion neurons (Herculano-Houzel, 2009). Moreover, some areas of the brain, like the hippocampus, can generate new neurons throughout life. The rate of renewal begins to slow when we are in the age range of our mid-sixties, and the number of neurons we lose begins to outweigh the number of neurons we create. In young adults thousands of new brain cells are born every day, although many of those die shortly after. In order to survive, these new brain cells rely on a protein called WnT3 that is released by other, already existing cells called astrocytes. While the number of neurons does not decrease substantially until the mid-sixties, some damage still occurs to the neurons over time, including the time from birth to adulthood. This cumulative damage occurs to the mitochondria, those organelle structures that supply the cell with energy in the form of ATP (adenosine triphosphate). Mitochondria wear out over time, which means that, while some neurons break down altogether, other neurons continue to work at a limited capacity.

Synaptic Plasticity (Strengthening of Synaptic Connections or Changes Thereof)

Synapses number in the trillions because they connect neurons in many ways. Each synapse needs continued maintenance, and is highly responsive to changes in the brain, which can then strengthen or weaken the synapse, cause it to dissipate, collapse, or even be rebuilt. For example, every time a word is encountered and processed, the connection of the record of that word is strengthened or modified. Exactly how the synapse is updated is discussed among neuroscientists. The discussion centers around the question as to whether the chemical process of updating relies on a self-regenerating network, as Routtenberg and Rekart (2005) explain, or if an individual synapse can update itself. With regard to processing words that involve several areas of the brain, including the synchronous firing of neurons, converging zones, and neuronal language circuits, the conclusion would seem to be that a network is required.

Something we must be aware of is that the life of a synapse is more adaptable than that of a neuron. A synapse can change. This is important, as the synapse holds the record of a word and that record can be recalled at any moment in time. It implies that new information can be added to the existing record, either linguistic information (i.e., another meaning to the same word) or non-linguistic information (i.e., another situation in which the word is encountered). Such adaptability is necessary to store the record of a word efficiently. Languages such as English or German have more than 100,000 words. However, most people are familiar with less than half of them, in the sense that they have heard them before. Actively using those words, most people have a vocabulary of less than 10 percent of 100,000 words. Let's assume you have 10,000 records of your first language stored in the non-mesial region in the form of synapses. Of course, the number goes up when acquiring another language. Still, in the grand scheme of things, storing that many records of words is very much achievable. After all, we have trillions of synapses in our brain.

When learning another language there are certain phases that specifically benefit the process of word acquisition. Our processing capacity continues to develop until we are in our mid-twenties, which according to some psychologists corresponds to the time when most memories are formed. The age before six is particularly important, because this is the time when children develop their vocabularies (between the age of six and eight, children know about 14,000 words), in addition to some of their language skills (listening, speaking). It has been argued, therefore, that children need to have the basic speaking skills developed before the age of six to eight (Korte, 2009; Lenneberg, 1967). They continue to develop those skills, as well as learning to read and write, at school. Between the ages of eleven and fourteen, they develop the ability to analyze abstractions and continue to develop the phonological loop (the loop is functioning by the age of six, but the interplay of rehearsal and temporary storage continues to develop until about sixteen). The process of coding words from encounter to long-term memory is refined and optimized until the mid-twenties (Korte, 2009). Synapses continue to form throughout all of these developmental phases. Their formation or modification is based on a series of biochemical reactions that run through the brain via the bloodstream. Growing up, some of these chemicals change, particularly hormones. We notice physical changes: around the age of six children start to grow significantly, around the age of eleven to fourteen the physical features change, and in the early twenties those features are refined. Naturally, changes also occur in the brain. We will discuss this in more detail in Chapter 5, "First and Second Language Acquisition." Apart from the fact that certain developmental phases are ideal for learning another language, much depends also on the situation in which the word is acquired, as well as when the word was used last.

For example, imagine you are twenty-five, and are traveling through Germany and need to buy a ticket. Before your trip you learned a few words including "Fahrkarte" [ticket]. You start your trip in Hamburg and are happy that at the train station the ticket salesperson understands you when you ask for a "Fahrkarte." You continue to use this word on your journey until you get to a small village in Bavaria, where suddenly no one seems to understand your request. Instead, they use "Bileddl" (local dialect for "ticket"). Through an exchange of gestures you finally realize that the two words actually mean the same thing. You travel a bit more through Bavaria and buy a few more "Bileddl," after which you return to Hamburg. At the train station you ask for a "Bileddl" and the person selling the tickets gives you a blank stare. In fact, if s/he speaks French, s/he might think you are French (the French word for a ticket is "billet"). To summarize your situation: you learned "Fahrkarte" first and used it more often than "Bileddl," but when you needed to say "Fahrkarte" what came to mind was "Bileddl," because that is the word you used most recently. The context or situation in which you learned "Bileddl" may have also contributed to the reason your brain recalled it over "Farhrkarte." Since the word "Bileddl" was not in the guidebook, you may have felt proud to learn it, especially in the somewhat emotional moment of your wild gestures. On the other hand, you were happy when the ticket agent in Hamburg understood you when you said "Fahrkarte." Therefore, which word you remember best may depend on how emotional you found each situation. This example shows the interplay of several factors when trying to recall a word in another language.

Now imagine you are sixty-five. Forty years after your trip to Germany, you visit the country again. There is one difference: when you went to Germany at the age of twenty-five, you only went to Hamburg, where you could use "Fahrkarte" – the word you had previously learned – without a problem. Over the years since then, you sometimes recalled the word "Fahrkarte" when asked about your trip. Now this time you do go to Bavaria and you are in the same situation described above: you must learn the word "Bileddl." This time in Hamburg, when you ask the ticket agent for another ticket, you will say "Fahrkarte." The reason for this has to do with age. Even though you used the word "Bileddl" a few times, and more recently than "Fahrkarte," the synapse around the word record of "Billedl" is still new in comparison, and therefore relatively fragile. Your brain will tend to select and recall the more established word record, in this case "Fahrkarte," which you learned at an earlier age and used more often. Once again, if the word is connected to an emotional experience at the time it is learned, the heightened sensory information adds to the strength of the synapse.

Somewhere between our mid-twenties and sixties, our body begins to slow down, and the aging process accelerates from our sixties and beyond. Of course, we can still form new synapses, but it does take more time for the aging brain to modify or create a new synapse. At the same time, existing synapses start to dissipate. The processes under which synapses dissipate continue throughout life, as do the processes in which new synapses are formed. However, although both processes continue, one slows down. When we get older, we actually lose more synapses than we can create. Why do synapses dissipate? One of the reasons has to do with maintenance. As we age, our body's production of neurotransmitters, proteins, and enzymes slows down and consequently the synapses cannot be properly replenished. For example, with age our bodies start to produce less dopamine and acetylcholine, two of the neurotransmitters that assist the modification or formation of new synapses (Scheibel, 1992). Furthermore, less myelin is produced (Aleman, 2013). Myelin is a protein that provides a sheath around the axon. Among other things, the sheath consists of lipids, including fats. These fats insulate the axon, which in turn results in greater acceleration of the signal. If less myelin is produced, signal transmission slows, and in some cases fades, before it even reaches the next neuron.

Naturally, if the word record has been built and reinforced in the manner of an eight-lane highway overpass, it will not fall apart as quickly as a log over a creek. Therefore, older people are often able to recall information that goes back to a time when they were young, since that information has been recalled numerous times over many years. This also explains why it is possible to recall words learned in another language (if the speaker acquired the second language in youth and has maintained it to some degree), but difficult to recall new words even in one's first language. For example, the modern word "selfie" has only come into the vocabulary of everyday speech recently. For an older person, whose synapse production and maintenance have slowed, a new word in the native language, such as "selfie," can be difficult to learn and to recall. If the speaker, in this case someone over the age of sixty-five, does not take photos of herself and upload them to a social media site or webpage, it is even less likely that s/he will create a record of that word. However, if the speaker takes "selfies" or simply uses the word frequently, s/he will learn that word regardless of age. It will take more time, as the word needs to be repeated more often compared to when one was younger. We discuss this in more detail in Chapter 5, "First and Second Language Acquisition," where we also learn if it is possible to learn a new language at an older age.

In terms of science and medicine, we must ask if the person's rate of synaptic decline occurs at a speed considered standard by researchers, or if a person's rate of synaptic decline is somewhat accelerated compared to others in the same age group, as a greater rate of decline may signify MCI. We must also check that the proteins and enzymes function properly, because improper protein and enzyme function can result in dementia. Alzheimer's disease, the most severe form of dementia, can attack and destroy the existing neurons and synapses.

In summary, every time we access a memory, a chemical process triggers and updates the synapse. If the synapse is not triggered or updated, it eventually dissipates. This will mean that the bridge that allows us to recall that specific memory is no longer available. The strength of the synapse depends on how the information was coded. The synapse can dissipate within months, years, or decades, depending on the strength of the record and the frequency of maintenance. To avoid a synapse dissipating and the word record becoming difficult to recall, the word must receive maintenance. It needs to be recalled. When we say that a modified or new synapse can provide permanent access to information and create a long-term memory, we must keep in mind that nothing is permanent. In particular, memory is not permanent. A synapse can gradually fall apart over time if the speaker no longer accesses that particular memory, or it can happen suddenly in the case of a stroke, injury, or accident that has caused damage to the brain.

In second language acquisition, the same faculties are used to process words forming a language network: the phonological loop, Broca's and Wernicke's areas, the hippocampus, the amygdala, and the cortices. Researchers discuss whether the neuroanatomical circuits developed in second language acquisition are the same or different to the circuits previously developed when the speaker acquired his or her first language. This may present a complex issue. Language acquisition depends on two main processes: the processing of words and the coding of grammar. In Chapter 1, "A New Word," Figure 2 showed how words and grammar are key components in communication. In general, there is reason to believe that the brain uses the same circuits as it processes words, whereas, when it processes grammar, the circumstances under which the L2 is/was acquired determines whether or not the same circuits are used. Such factors include the phase in life in which L2 was acquired, as well as the environment in which it was acquired; for example, whether or not the language acquired continues to be spoken in that environment. Naturally, the process of word recall must involve speed, because when we wish to use a word we must recall it quickly. Speed depends on the proficiency of the speaker, as well as on his or her motivation and preferences. We will discuss this in more detail in Chapters 5 and 6, "First and Second Language Acquisition" and "The Bilingual Lexicon and Speaker."

4 Cognitive Load

Cognitive Demand

In second language acquisition, researchers often analyze how often words occur in a text. They also investigate word associations or modes of presentation. In contrast, few studies have been carried out to research words at the microlevel, that is, the components of words, such as lexemes and phonemes, and how these components are acquired when learning another language. In order to facilitate the learning of words, it is very helpful to know how these lexemes and phonemes are processed. When learners acquire new words with the assistance of word games, association trees, or other types of input, we need to ask two questions: What is actually being processed? How much of that can our memory handle?

As mentioned, learning 5,000 words in another language allows us to communicate in most situations (Schmitt, 2010b). The challenge is to acquire those words in a short period of time and to sustain the acquisition. Surveying university language programs, Milton (2009) reports that it is surprising how little students know in terms of active vocabulary after having studied another language for two years. Active vocabulary refers to the ability to recall a word from memory. One line of investigation analyzes optimal spacing patterns; that is, the repetition of words in specific intervals within a specific time frame. This has been tried in education and cognitive psychology, as well as in neuroscience. However, before we go into detail as to how studies in this area are carried out in Chapter 7, "Spacing," we need to learn more about memory itself.

Learning another language there are two larger systems: vocabulary and grammar (see Figure 2 in Chapter 1, "A New Word"). Every learner not only faces the challenge of how to acquire many new words but to acquire a set of rules as to how those words are grammatically coded and put together into a proper sentence. In his model of what it means to know a word (see Chapter 1, "A New Word"), Nation (2001) distinguishes between form (spoken/written) and meaning (concepts/relationships). The questions he raises are how form and meaning interact, what parts of a word are needed in order to recognize or produce a word, and what other words the word is associated with. With regard to the relationship of form to meaning, the question is how phonemes and lexemes are matched when processing words.

Analyzing the development and behavior of systems, the dynamic systems model provides some insight. The model was developed in mathematics and stresses the point that information processes do not necessarily follow a clear, linear path. It can rather be seen as a dynamic activity with many variables that interact and change over time (Miller, 2002). In this way, the model attempts to describe the flow of relationships among the components of some whole phenomenon (Thomas, 2001). It assumes that systems are self-organizing, and has been applied to second language acquisition by various researchers (de Bot, Lowie, and Verspoor, 2007; Larsen-Freeman, 1997; Larsen-Freeman and Cameron, 2008; Spivey, 2008; van Geert, 1991, 2008).

There are four core concepts: two are related to development and two to behavior. First, development is dynamic. The current state of a system depends on its prior states and is the starting point for future states (Thelen, 2005). Second, the components of a system interact with one another and form patterns. If a component changes, it impacts other components of the system (Thomas, 2001). Third, behavior is both flexible and stable. While organisms evolve they attempt to find a state of relative stability known as the "preferred state" (Miller, 2002). Fourth, behavior depends on the person's individual skills and motivation (Spencer et al., 2006).

We can apply these concepts to the acquisition of words. We try to build our vocabulary over time. First, the number of words we know at any given point in time is based on the prior number of words we have attempted to acquire. Each attempt might lead to successful acquisition. Our current number of attempts is linked to the success rate of acquiring a word. This is not a one-to-one relation; we need several attempts to acquire one word. Once a word is acquired we have time to acquire another word, which in turn might also need several attempts. Second, we have to decode and encode words because we usually speak in sentences. We need to know the grammatical forms a word can take. The two systems of vocabulary and grammar interact and can positively and negatively impact each other depending on the cognitive demand (we discuss this in more detail in the next paragraph). Third, we forget words we have previously acquired. Yet, we can reacquire those words, and in that sense our vocabulary evolves in a non-linear way. Fourth, each of us tries to build a vocabulary s/he is happy with. This vocabulary differs from learner to learner in size and type depending on the learner's motivation. Some of us are happy with knowing fewer words as long as we get the message across, others like to have a vocabulary of thousands of words. The words we acquire often represent our interest and learning situation. If we are interested in traveling, we try to build a vocabulary around greetings, making reservations, food and drinks, sightseeing, and activities one can do. If we are interested in cooking, we try to learn more words related to food than other learners might do.

Testing the theory, Robinson and Mervis (1998) carried out a study on lexical growth in children in relation to the correct use of plural forms. Their study showed a negative relation between the two systems of vocabulary learning and grammatical encoding: in times when many new words were acquired, children made little gains in the acquisition of correct plural forms; whereas when more and more plural forms were used correctly, fewer new words were acquired. The two systems competed with one another. It's a good example for demonstrating that resources in our mind are limited. It fits well into Nation's (2001) distinction of form and meaning and how they interact. First, phonemes and lexemes need to be matched, then morphemes identified or encoded. If morphemes do not fit the word selected for speech production, the matching process might have to start again. This places additional demand on the cognitive system. If the demand is too high, the system has to choose between one or the other.

For children acquiring their first language, the language system is still developing. Therefore, the development of vocabulary and grammar is more predictable in the first few years until they begin to acquire strategies at the age of eight. At that point individual preferences start playing more of a role. We learn more about the phases of language development in Chapter 5, "First and Second Language Acquisition." For adults acquiring a second language the situation is different. They can draw on their knowledge of language as a system. Still, their vocabulary and grammar of the language they are learning needs to develop. However, as they have developed a system already, individual preferences are a key factor. While some learners are happy to use words in their speech even if they are grammatically incorrect, others only use words if they have been encoded properly. It needs to be mentioned, however, that once a threshold is passed – that is, a certain number of words have been acquired – the development of both systems go hand in hand for children and adults alike.

Attention

In Chapter 2, "Memory, Language, and the Brain," we learned that the main component of working memory is the so-called central executive that directs, divides, and switches attention to incoming words, a process that demands much energy (Baddeley, 2007). Postle (2006) suggests that attention causes the brain to light up the faculties of working memory, which then zoom in on the incoming information, which in turn sets off the process of rehearsal. The frontal lobe of our brain, where the central executive is located, is a region that in general is associated with planning, organization, and decision-making

(Baddeley, 2007). The cognitive demand of processing new words is high, and resources linked to attention compete against each other as the limited capacity model outlines (Skehan, 1998, 2009a; Skehan and Foster, 2001). Since resources are limited, if a word cannot be processed in time, it falls out of the loop to make room for a new word, but this process also depends on whether the incoming information is new or already known. If a known word is processed, less attention is required than with a new, unfamiliar word. The demand linked to attention impacts to what degree a word is processed and to what degree we know a word (Nation, 2001). If we know all or only parts of the word's form and meaning, this in turn affects the recall of a word and thereby the fluency, accuracy, and complexity of speech.

The three factors – fluency, accuracy, and complexity – are part of the key goals of speech production (Skehan, 1998; Skehan and Foster, 1997). Fluency refers to the speed with which we can recall words from memory; accuracy, to the recall of the correct words, grammatically coded with the correct morphemes; and complexity refers to the number and variety of words stored, including those with highly intricate lexemes. A word with a strong record can be recalled faster than a word with a fragile record. In order to recall a word with a fragile record, much discrimination has to take place to sort out all the lexemes and phonemes that differentiate it from any similar words. It is important to note that to recall a word with more speed does not automatically mean to recall it with more accuracy. As Skehan (2009a) argues, since our capacity to process information is limited, more attention on content often means less attention is available to process form. It can happen that a word is recalled quickly and is pronounced with the correct combination of a lexeme to its phonemes, but with an incorrect morpheme. Skehan (2012) refers to this as a trade-off: if you focus on one aspect, the other aspects might be neglected.

An example from the many language courses I have taught is that learners of German whose first language is English often have difficulties with plural forms of nouns. Talking about movies, they recall "Film" [movie] and pronounce it correctly but use an incorrect plural such as "Filmen" instead of "Filme." The reason for this has to do with the way morphemes are processed in speech production. A lexeme is recorded with morphological markers but not actual morphemes. These markers function as placeholders. They indicate what type of morpheme can be linked to the lexeme. The actual morpheme is attached to the lexeme later. By saying "Filmen" instead of "Filme," the speech is not only inaccurate but fluency is also compromised, as the mistake has to be corrected, which takes time.

We need to consider that what kind of trade-off is being made depends on the level of proficiency of the speaker as well as his or her individual preferences (Cook and Singleton, 2014; Singleton, 1995, 2007). A beginning learner of another language often has to decide what is more important: to get the message across by quickly recalling words even if they are not in the correct grammatical form, or to assemble a perfect sentence which may take extra time. This can also be a problem when the language learner recalls the lexeme of a word, because the concept of a word that is tied to the lexeme in one language might be different in another language. We will return to that issue and learn more about proficiency levels in Chapter 6, "The Bilingual Lexicon and Speaker." Essentially, a speaker has to make a decision whether or not the word s/he chooses to recall expresses what s/he wants to say. Naturally the trade-off between fluency and accuracy also influences complexity of speech, as a beginning second language speaker can decide to stick with simple sentences, since, at beginning proficiency, the cognitive demand is so high that not enough attention can be given to all three factors at once. With an increase in proficiency, the three factors of fluency, accuracy, and complexity will also start to complement each other. For example, a speaker with a large number of previously acquired words at his or her disposal can more quickly vary the word order in a sentence, which will in turn make the sentence more complex without sacrificing fluency.

Cognitive demand has been linked to issues of automaticity (Schmidt, 2001). Automaticity refers to the phenomena that the more something is repeated, the less effort it requires. This can have positive or negative effects. When we learn a new word, "elaborate rehearsal" is required (Craik and Lockhart, 1972). The phonemes and lexeme of the word need to be identified and a record of the word created. In this situation, automaticity has a negative effect. Less effort reduces the need for cognitive attention and less attention can lead to mistakes or the possibility that the word might not be processed sufficiently. If we assume that the phonological loop rehearses the phonemes each time we repeat a word, we may try to learn a new word by repeating it several times in a row. However, this method may prove unsuccessful because the loop can hold information for up to two minutes. The trace of a word fades after half a second or, if prolonged via the temporary store, after about two seconds, but the word is still available for processing for a minute or two longer (Tranel and Damasio, 2002). It means that the second repetition overlaps with the first, which in turn means that no additional attention is given to the word and the word only receives attention once, when it is first encountered. The question then is, how long the pause between each repetition should be. As we saw in the example of *Aplysia*, it remembered its reaction for up to a day when stimulated repeatedly with no pauses in between but up to a month when stimulated with pauses. Does this imply that there should be at least a day in between repetitions? Research showed that during sleep our brain reviews the day's information. We return to that issue in Chapter 7, "Spacing." It should be noted, though, that once a word has been acquired and can be processed automatically, it has a positive effect on learning more new words because it frees up space in the phonological loop. Rehearsal of words that are known to the speaker is referred to as "maintenance rehearsal" (Craik and Lockhart, 1972). If we hear a sentence that has a word in it we have never heard before, but we do know all of the other words, we can focus on that one new word.

Studies have shown a delay of up to 100 milliseconds from the time we encounter a word until the time our brain begins to process it in the language faculties such as the loop or Wernicke's area (for a summary of this issue, see Pulvermüller, 2000). Pulvermüller argues that this is quite surprising given that communication depends on processing information quickly. A possible explanation lies in the demand placed on our cognitive attention whenever we encounter a new word, and in particular when we process several words at a time. Fortunately, switching attention from one word to another does not require much extra effort (Allport, Styles, and Hsieh, 1994). Unfortunately, a word that receives twice the amount of attention than another word does not double its chance that the process of "elaborative rehearsal" will be complete, because the ratio of word processing to cognitive attention is not one-to-one. If we were to increase the number of words (or non-words or digits, which are often used in these studies) processed simultaneously during a task, this would increase the difficulty of the task and decrease the rate of recall (Logie et al., 2004). Rolke et al. (2001) found that if words are presented in rapid succession – that is, the time between the end of the previous word and the beginning of the following word is very short (250 milliseconds) – participants only remember half of the words presented on a list. The participants must simply skip some words, because there is not enough time for the loop to rehearse and temporarily store words. Asked after the test if they remembered those missing words, most participants had no idea that those words had actually been on the list.

Processing Problems

Acquiring a new word, the process of matching a word's phonemes to its lexeme is fragile (Baddeley, Gathercole, and Papagno, 1998). Phonemes must be discriminated against other phonemes during rehearsal in the loop. The loop compares new phonemes to phonemes that are known and called up from Wernicke's area. At the same time, lexemes are called up from the non-mesial region to assist identifying the incoming word. The form-to-meaning relationship needs to be established (Nation, 2001) and a record of that created. Calling up lexemes from the non-mesial region in order to utter a word and match the proper phonemes to the word to be pronounced is a process during which errors can occur.

This process often presents a challenge to young children. At the age of two to three, children create all kinds of words. The child might say "bathmup" instead of "bathtub." Those word creations do not last very long, though.

Eventually, the child will code the phonemes and lexeme correctly. We will return to that in Chapter 5, “First and Second Language Acquisition.” Studying the word processes of children who were just about to enter primary school, Gathercole and Baddeley (1989) investigated the ability of such children to repeat non-words, since to process a non-word relies on the rehearsal of phonemes, in particular on temporary storage. The children, ages four and five, were asked to simply repeat back non-words that were read to them. The non-words varied in length from one to four syllables. Gathercole and Baddeley had run other tests with the children to determine the size of their vocabulary knowledge at that time, as well as their reading skills. Only children with normal vocabulary scores and who could not read yet were analyzed. This was done so the non-words chosen would not resemble any of the known words and children with the ability to read would not be able to figure out a link between a non-word and an existing word. Children were retested one, two, and four years later, and at that time their vocabulary scores were also tested. Results showed that the ability to repeat non-words at the age of four helped children to develop a large vocabulary. Those children who had low non-word repetition scores also had low vocabulary scores in the follow-up tests one, two, and four years later.

Studies such as this show the importance of the phonological loop for learning new words at a young age. Ellis (1996) argues that the ability to repeat phonological sequences is crucial for word learning: when acquiring words in another language a learner needs to code and decode those sequences of phonemes as well as match them with lexemes and morphemes. He also acknowledges that individual differences among children might play a larger role than we think. The phonological loop develops over time and, although the brain’s rehearsal and temporary storage areas function well by the age of six, the rehearsal processes are further refined until the age of sixteen. As children develop at different rates, so does their phonological loop. Researchers continue to carry out studies that investigate the role of the phonological loop in children who learn a second language. In Finland, Service (1992) tested nine-year-old elementary school children by asking them to repeat back unfamiliar English sounds. These children did not know English yet, but they began to learn English a couple of weeks later. Service found that those children who had good scores in the repeat-back task scored higher on an English vocabulary test given two and a half years later than those children who had low scores. In fact, as early as 1966, Baddeley (1966c) proposed that temporary storage is useful in an early learning phase. When children are faced with the challenge of learning many new words, they may rely on the temporary storage in addition to the rehearsal. Later on, they rely less and less on storage as they develop semantic networks to help them process words. When adults learn new words, the situation is a bit more complex. If the new word has a semantic connection to another word that is already known to the learner and s/he can establish that connection, temporary storage may not be needed. If the word has no connection and is literally new, it will be needed. This is why beginning language learners who acquire an L2 at first rely heavily on the transfer from their L1.

In summary, studies (Baddeley, Gathercole, and Papagno, 1998; Ellis, 1996; Service, 1992) have shown that processing problems in the phonological loop impact the acquisition of learning new words in another language.

The difficulty of processing depends on the complexity of the word as well as how much of the word is known already. The complexity depends on several factors:

- number of syllables (word length)
- similarity (in meaning [lexemes], pronunciation [phonemes], both (lexemes and phonemes)
- emotional connotations/situations (emotional words).

These factors are linked to a word's memory trace. Phonemes and lexemes have their own individual traces that fade quickly (known as trace decay) if not renewed (Baddeley, 2007). If it fades, phonemes or lexemes cannot be discriminated against each other. We will return to this issue later in this chapter.

The first factor relates to how many phonemes need to be processed. This is known as the effect of word length. Baddeley and his colleagues tested this effect as early as 1975. They showed that longer words are more difficult to remember because there are more syllables to process. This presents a challenge, given the limited amount of time the brain has to process a word before the memory trace disappears. The effect is extremely robust, as Baddeley reports, after testing it many times (Baddeley, 2007). We might ask if there is anything that can be done about long words? After all, the trace disappears every time the word is rehearsed. The best strategy seems to be to rehearse the components of the word, since longer words tend to be made up of compounds. Let's imagine ourselves once again at the airport in Frankfurt. We must now pick up our luggage from the baggage carousel. We need to find a sign that says, "Gepäckausgabe," meaning "luggage claim." "Gepäck" is "luggage" and "Ausgabe" is "distribution." In this example, the compound word is made up of two nouns, but compounds can be constructed of nouns, verbs, adjectives, prefixes, suffixes, or any combination of these.

The second factor is similarity. If the lexeme of a new word is similar to that of a known word, it is easily identified. If these words are from two different languages, they are called cognates. A speaker who uses cognates to build up his or her vocabulary will more quickly acquire the second language. Most people who do not speak German still understand words such as "Familie," "Bier," or "Automobil." However, one must still be cautious, as a word with a similar lexeme in both L1 and L2 might still differ somewhat in its concept, as we explored in the example of "Kaffee." In addition, we must consider whether the sequence of phonemes of a new word is similar to that of another word, such as "Reihe" [line/row] and "Reise" [journey/travel]. The only difference between the two is the second syllable "h" vs. "s." If so, this can pose problems, since, in order to distinguish between two words, the phonemes of each must be discriminated against the other. If the phonemes are similar, it will take more time to discriminate between them. This is known as the effect of phonological similarity. It had been tested as early as 1966 when Baddeley (1966a, 1966b) showed that words with similar sounds are more difficult to recall. For example, it is more difficult to remember word lists such as "cat, map, man, hat, mat" than to remember word lists such as "pit, day, cow, pen, hot" (examples taken from Baddeley). Baddeley tested this with native speakers, but the same problem persists in L2. Therefore, when we attempt to acquire words in another language we should not rehearse words of similar sounds within the same learning session. Words such as "Reihe" and "Reise" should be rehearsed in different lessons. If we repeat the phonologically similar words several times, however, the effect disappears, because each rehearsal process discriminates between some of the phonemes until, with enough repetitions, they are all discriminated.

The third factor relating to the complexity of processing words conveys that words with an emotional connotation are processed differently than regular words. Emotional words are processed with heightened activation, which results in a strong record, as described in Chapter 3, "Synaptic Connections." Emotional words activate the senses, which release more serotonin, dopamine, or acetylcholine and assist in the formation or modification of a synapse. Moreover, emotional words are often associated with a particular situation or an event. Remember when you burned your tongue drinking "heißer Kaffee" at Frankfurt airport? Part of the record of this emotional situation included words. This leads us to ask whether only emotional words such as "heiß" can be fast-tracked, or if non-emotional words such as "Kaffee" associated with an emotional event can also be fast-tracked? This has been recently studied and we will return to that in Chapter 8, "Word Analysis."

What is important is that all these factors – word length, phonological similarity, emotional connotation – influence whether or not our brain will create a strong record of the word. They are particularly important for content words. In general, content words such as nouns, verbs, adjectives, and some adverbs carry independent meaning (Aitchison, 2003). They have a rich lexeme that expresses a concept via the lemma and they have bound or system morphemes. Content words make up a high percentage of the overall words in a given language, which therefore increases the odds that some of them will fit the characteristics of longer words and words that are similar in sound. The rich lexemes of content words can also express emotion. Function words, on the other hand, such as prepositions, conjunctions, fillers, articles, and some adverbs, are simpler. They do not carry independent meaning and only function together with content words. Naturally, words such as prepositions or articles do not have an emotional connotation. The number of function words in a language is quite limited; therefore similarities are less likely to occur. Furthermore, function words also tend to be short.

There is reason to believe that our brains process function words in a different way than content words. Some evidence comes from studies with non-words. The workings of the subvocal rehearsal and the temporary storage as part of the phonological loop are key components when it comes to processing new words. Many studies, in particular by Vallar and Papagno (1993, 2002; Papagno and Vallar, 1992,), as well as by Gathercole and Baddeley (1989, 1990), have investigated the exact relationship between these two components. These studies tested the workings of the phonological loop by using words, non-words, syllables or nonsense syllables, or digits. Usually, participants were asked to recall as many items as possible after a time delay. Non-words are particularly interesting because, unlike words, they do not have a lexeme that can be easily identified. Consequently the rehearsal process relies on prolonged time in the temporary storage in order to correctly identify the phonemes. Testing non-words is therefore a good indicator of whether the phonological loop functions properly. In general, when we study the actual process of coding at the phonemic level, it is useful to take away the cues to isolate the phonemes. Several studies show that non-words are more difficult to recall than words. One of the most comprehensive studies on this topic was conducted by Gathercole et al. (2001). They presented undergraduate students at the University of Bristol with lists of words and lists of non-words. The words and non-words were one-syllable combinations of consonant-vowel-consonant (CVC). On recognition – a list was presented once and then another list was presented that had either the same or a different word order – there was no difference. Words and non-words were recognized with the same degree of accuracy. The design of the study accounts for this: when researchers presented the student with a second-word list shortly after the first, rehearsal of the phonemes was still in progress within the loop. Because the lexeme had not yet been identified, the variable of word or non-word made no difference to the rehearsal process. On recall, however, students remembered words with more accuracy than non-words. On the recall test, researchers spoke the words to the students and asked them to repeat back the CVC sequences. The number of CVC sequences increased with each list and researchers measured the point at which the number of CVC sequences increased beyond the students' ability to recall them accurately. The process of recall in part explains why the students found it more difficult to recall non-words than words. In order to recall a word, the phonemes must be put in order, a process that is easier to do if they can be matched to a lexeme. Notably, the study shows the importance of the interplay of phonemes and lexemes. Due to the fact that recall took place right after the students viewed (or heard) the words or non-words, no record of the word was created. Nevertheless, in the case of whether or not the student could recall a word over a non-word, the presence of a lexeme made the difference. This, in turn, seems to show the advantage of content words over function words.

Another interesting study in this area comes from the University of Wales, where Speciale, Ellis, and Bywater (2004) carried out two experiments. In the first experiment, undergraduate students with no knowledge of German as a foreign language learned twenty-four German words. For each word, the English word was presented visually and the German equivalent heard on audio twice. This was done twice, so German words were heard four times in total. Two tests were carried out: first, a test on production, which showed the English words in random order and asked students to say the German word; and second, a test on comprehension, where students listened to the German words in random order and typed the English equivalent into a box on a computer screen. In a second experiment, students listened to non-words of two, three, or four syllables eight times and had to indicate each time whether they heard the preceding non-word in the list. The researchers measured the students' success by how fast they remembered all non-words, as well as by how many syllables of the non-words they could correctly repeat. Results showed that the ability to repeat non-words was positively correlated to the ability to produce a German word. However, it had no impact on the ability to recognize a German word. The importance of the lexeme when processing a new word explains this difference, and in fact gives indirect evidence as to how the process functions. When we recall a word in another language, in particular when prompted by the equivalent word in our first language, the records of words are activated in the non-mesial region. The focus is on the lexemes that are matched to phonemes. When we simply hear a word in another language, our brain relies more on processing phonemes before these are matched to lexemes, even in the case of a word that we have heard several times before.

If function words are processed differently, the question is how to acquire them. Using spacing intervals, is there an advantage to using one type of interval over the other? Is that linked to the number of rehearsals? We will answer these questions in Chapter 8, "Word Analysis."

We need to remember that processing a new word is fluid and dynamic and relies on underlying neural processes that bind the acoustic representation of a word (Buchsbaum and D'Esposito, 2008). The description of the loop with its two subsystems of rehearsal and temporary storage seems static. However, if it were as static as it is described in the explanation of working memory, it would be less likely to make mistakes, because everything would be perfectly compartmentalized. However, we all make mistakes when we speak, not just in a new language but also in the language we first learned, our L1. Most often we make mistakes when we try to recall a word; for example, we switch words or mispronounce them. This is a matter of serial order, which we will discuss further in the following section.

Speech Errors

Initially the loop was thought to be able to process only few words over a period of seconds. However, it is now believed that the loop can process up to ten words and hold them for up to one or two minutes with the use of the temporary storage (Tranel and Damasio, 2002). This discovery concerns the memory trace of each word. In fact, each phoneme and lexeme has its individual memory trace, that is, the rate at which they fade, known as trace decay. The traces are of different duration. To process a word involves something like organized chaos, where phonemes and the lexeme are in varying stages of being processed. The actual trace lasts for half a second or less, though the interplay of rehearsal and storage can prolong the trace for up to two seconds. The memory trace itself is very fragile, particularly the first time a word is encountered. In most cases, we must encounter a word several times before our brain creates a record of the word. Likewise, repeated encounters of the word lead to the modification or creation of a new synapse. If we encounter a word several times, and if our brain subsequently creates or modifies a synapse, then the trace of the word's phonemes and lexeme will become more stable.

Our brain can reactivate words and rehearse them again, even if they have been put aside in the phonological loop's storage subsystem, as long as the trace of the word's phonemes and lexeme remains accessible. This implies that rehearsal of the same word in intervals – that is, with a time delay in between rehearsals – might lead to more successful processing. Until the early 1990s, most researchers assumed that, once the trace was gone, it could not be recovered. Since then, however, some researchers such as Cowan (1992, 1993) argued that the memory trace does not necessarily fade away completely. When we process a new word the challenge is to rehearse it concurrently with the next incoming word. This explains part of the function of the temporary storage: to make room for more words in the phonological loop. However, Cowan argued that there are small pauses – of milliseconds – between each word, during which the loop scans the new incoming word. In a study with forty-four children aged four and five who recalled word lists (words were spoken at a rate of one second per word to the children, who had to recall them orally), Cowan measured the time required for the child to pronounce a word, as well as the time the child needed to recall all of the words. Researchers debated whether the ability to pronounce a word quickly in order to make room for the next word could increase memory capacity. Cowan found no correlation.

Results from children with excellent scores on the number of items recalled correctly (four or five items) used the same amount of time per word as children who had low scores (two items). However, Cowan also found that children with excellent scores overall required more time to recall all of the words. Although it is logical to expect that the child would require additional time to pronounce four or five words compared to two, the question was how the brain of these children was able to recall all of those words. The brain of the higher-scoring children may have scanned the words in the small pauses between words (because the pronunciation length of each word was measured), which would have allowed them to reactivate a word that had not yet been rehearsed. Cowan's research thus implies that even a word encountered for the first time is available for rehearsal for more than two seconds, and in fact for up to two minutes. Exactly how the brain uses the pause to scan a word is unclear. Based on these and other experiments, Cowan (1999) suggests that the central executive of working memory scans words constantly, regardless of whether they are currently processed or not. It does so by directing, dividing, and switching attention. The function of the central executive, according to Cowan, is not only to decide which words are processed immediately when we encounter them but also to keep the words that are not attended to immediately in a holding pattern. This happens before the phonological loop starts its process. Therefore, in theory, it might be possible for several words to be processed in the loop (some are rehearsed in the loop while others are temporarily stored in the subsystem) and for several other words to be in a holding pattern in the central executive.

Speech errors provide an insight into how phonemes, lexemes, and morphemes interact. They have been researched for decades and different classifications and models have been proposed (for an overview, see Aitchison, 1992). Speech errors are not random, but are either a question of incorrect selection or incorrect assemblage, as Fromkin (1973) postulated some time ago. We can distinguish between lexical, phonological, and matching errors. As Dell and Reich (1981) explain, lexical errors can occur as a result of misordering a word (placing a word ahead of another word in a sentence), substituting a word, or blending two words into one. Phonological errors occur as a result of anticipating, preserving, or exchanging phonemes. Phonological errors follow rules. For example, "slips of the tongue" is sometimes mispronounced "stips of the lung" but not "tlip of the sung" (Fromkin, 1973). In English, the phonemes [s] and [l] and [s] and [t] can be paired to form the initial sound (at the beginning of a word), whereas the phonemes [t] and [l] cannot. Most interesting when investigating the interplay of phonemes, lexemes, and morphemes, however, are the type of speech errors that are a combination of incorrect processing of phonological and lexical information. These are called matching errors.

In order for speech to be produced, phonemes rehearsed in the phonological loop and matched to a lexeme in Broca's area must be aligned in the right order, known as serial order. A tag that is part of the record of a word and indicates the acceptable combination of phonemes to the lexeme helps to align the phonemes.

We make plenty of errors when we speak. To return to the scene at the airport in Frankfurt, we may say the following in order to ask for a coffee: "Einen Kaffee mit zwei Stück Zucker, bitte!" [A coffee with two pieces of sugar, please!] In German, "Stück Zucker" refers to "sugar cubes." Although these days sugar cubes are used less when ordering a coffee, as they have been replaced with small prepackaged sugar bags, in German sugar is still quantified by the number of pieces when ordering a beverage. If we are tired after a long flight, we may confuse the word for "sugar" with the word for "tea" and instead say: "Einen Kaffee mit zwei Stück Tee, bitte!" [A coffee with two pieces of tea, please!] This is a lexical substitution error. Interestingly enough, over three quarters of all such errors are within the same word class: for example, a noun is exchanged or mistaken for another noun. In this example, the sentence is grammatically correct but tea is ordered instead of sugar. So the meaning of the word is replaced. When the executive control recalled the lexeme of "Zucker" from the non-mesial region, lexemes of other things that are sweet or are used with sugar, such as "Tee," were simultaneously activated. The lexeme of "Tee" received more activation than the one for "Zucker." You might also say "Einen Zucker mit zwei Stück Kaffee, bitte!" [A sugar with two pieces of coffee, please!] This is a lexical misordering error. The lexemes for "Kaffee" and "Zucker" were both processed correctly; that is, the phonemes were matched to the proper lexeme and both words were activated. However, anticipating when the words were put into a sentence in the pre-speech plan, the fully processed word "Zucker" jumped ahead of the fully processed word "Kaffee." Or you say "Einen Kaffee mit zwei Stucker, bitter!" [A coffee with two pugar, please!]. "Stucker" is a combination of "Stück" and "Zucker." The two words have been blended into one. Incorrectly. The word "Stucker" does not make sense. The lexemes of "Stück" and "Zucker" were both processed fully; that is, they were recalled, discriminated from other lexemes and the phonemes matched to them. However, in the pre-speech plan they merged.

What causes these lexical errors? Why are lexemes not activated enough (word substitution) or the ones that are activated jump ahead or merge? It's a matter of attention. The central executive of working memory directs, divides, and switches attention (Baddeley, 2007) when encountering words as well as when recalling them. When substituting a word, attention is directed toward another lexeme. Errors in the pre-speech plan occur when attention is directed toward other parts of the sentence as the words have been processed fully. This allows words to jump ahead or merge. We do this when we are either tired (arriving at the airport in Frankfurt after a long flight) or distracted.

Let us once again return to the airport in Frankfurt. We have our coffee, but now it is time to find our luggage. We want to say:

"Mein Gepäck, bitte!" [My luggage, please!]

Instead, we say:

"Mein Gebäck, bitte!" [My cookies, please!]

This is a phonological error: "b" was switched for "p." In this case, it caused us to say another word with an entirely new meaning. The form-to-meaning relationship is intact because in producing the word "Gebäck" the lexeme of "Gebäck" was matched with its phonemes. "b" and "p" are both bilabial plosives. In the phonetic chart, they are next to each other. To explain such errors we can use Page and Norris's (1998) model. Page and Norris argue for a two-layer system of word nodes and phonemic nodes. Each word has a node for each phoneme and each phoneme has nodes itself. The word nodes represent the frame the phonemes operate in for a particular word; the phonemic nodes, the actual sounds. Dell (1988) first proposed the theory of a two-layer system where each phoneme carries an encoded node that tags the position of the phoneme, as well as associate nodes. The associate nodes are variations of the phoneme. A phoneme's position refers to whether it is the first, second, third, etc. phoneme of the word. A simple example in English is that "z" at the beginning of a word can only be followed by a vowel or "y' " but not by a consonant. Strings of nodes form that makes it easier to recall the word. In order to facilitate recall, in the string the first node links to the second node, the second to the third node, etc. Each node has to go through a filter that decides if the node is a match. If so, the node passes the filter and takes first position. If not, another node is brought up. In that sense, the previously encoded associate nodes help to find the correct node. Page and Norris call this competitive queuing. The string of nodes and the filter they have to pass through determine serial order. In the example above, "b" was switched for "p" because an associate node mistakenly received a boost as it traveled through the filter.

We might ask why an associate node mistakenly receives a boost. In general, these errors happen when we try to speak too fast, so a node goes through the filter unchecked. However, it is clear that we still need more details to fully understand errors such as "Gebäck" instead of "Gepäck." We know that the filter is not part of the record of a word. It has to operate independently to fulfill its function. What about the nodes of each phoneme? Phonemes are stored separately, which suggests that the nodes are not part of the record, either. In English, the range of phonemes is between 36 and 48, depending on the type of English spoken (for example, British English, American English, Australian English), plus 7 to 10 diphthongs. The combinations of phonemes are limited and there are rules as to which sequences are allowed and which sequences are not. With regard to the lexeme, however, we assume that the tag is part of the record. Does the tag, which indicates an acceptable combination of the lexeme to phonemes, include the initial phonemic node? If so, that would indeed be efficient. In the phoneme, the initial encoded node determines the phoneme's variations. Since phonemes and their variations are limited in number, there is no reason for the associate nodes to be part of the record. When we recall the initial phoneme with its first node, it is possible that associates are lined up by default.

Explaining the phonological similarity effect with the help of Page and Norris's (1998) model is a matter of too much competition. Here, the strings of nodes of phonemes are too similar to be discriminated in time before the word frame decays. With regard to word length, there may be too many phonemes to put in the correct order. There is not a lot of detail in the model to explain this further, so we will have to see if future research can shed some light on this issue.

With Page and Norris's (1998) model we can also explain, to a point, matching errors – that is, type of errors that are a combination of incorrect processing of phonological and lexical information.

Imagine we are back at the airport:

a) "Einen Kfafee mit zwei Stück Zucker, bitte!" [cfofee with two pieces of sugar, please!]

or

b) Einen Affkee mit zwei Stück Zucker, bitte!" [A offcee with two pieces of sugar, please!]

or

c) "Einen Chavee mit zwei Stück Zucker, bitte!" [A kovee with two pieces sugar, please!]

or

d) "Einen Achvee mit zwei Stück Zucker, bitte!" [An okvee with two pieces of sugar, please!]

In all of these examples, the words that replace "Kaffee" do not make sense. The form-to-meaning relationship is broken. The number of syllables usually remains constant, though, meaning the replacement word has the same number of syllables as the word one was looking for. In examples a) and b), the phonemes for "Kaffee" are not in the correct order. The difference between example a) and example b) is that the error in example a) is more likely to be made by adults, as adults often go by the first letter of a word, meaning they try to keep that sound in its place at the beginning of a word (the "K" for "Kaffee").

The error in example b) is more likely to be made by children, as children have enough to do focusing on the number of syllables. Word recall is a complex process that takes years to fully develop. While the phonological loop is functional by the age of six, the interplay of rehearsal to temporary storage is not refined until the age of sixteen. For children to practice rehearsal, it is easier to account for the number of syllables at the time of recall, but to figure out the correct order of the phonemes, rather than try to do both at once. Adult second language learners already know how language works as a system. However, when it comes to pronunciation they face the same challenge as children listening to the speech stream of their first language. They have to sort out the phonemes of the language they are learning. Therefore, these types of errors are not entirely uncommon in the initial phase of learning a second language. With a higher level of proficiency, adult second language learners will attempt to keep the sound of first letter of the word in place. Skehan (2009b) argues that trade-off effects likely occur when lexemes are matched to phonemes and encoded with morphemes. Most learners focus on the lexeme. As a result the word might be mispronounced or not grammatically encoded. When we mispronounce a word, the phonemes were either matched correctly to the lexeme but the prosody and coarticulation is out of sync, or the phonemes were assembled and aligned incorrectly so serial order is out of place.

We can explain the errors in examples a) and b) with Page and Norris's (1998) model. In that model, the phonemic nodes and word nodes interact. When we process a word, it receives an activation boost. While the word frame fills with the phonemes, one node receives a stronger boost than usual and jumps the queue to pass through the filter ahead of another node, thereby changing the order. Saying "Chavee" instead of "Kaffee" means that associated nodes received a stronger boost but they did not jump the queue, whereas in "Achvee" two things happened: the associated nodes received a stronger boost and they jumped the queue.

Whenever a phoneme is activated, similar-sounding phonemes are activated as well. In the examples, the sound of the word is replaced. In examples c) and d), "ch" replaced "k" because in German "ch" is sometimes pronounced as "k," and "v" replaced "f" because they are both labiodental fricatives, which means they are phonologically related.

In order to explain examples c) and d), we can use a model proposed by Burgess and Hitch (1999). There are some similarities to Page and Norris's (1998) model. In Burgess and Hitch's (1999) model are two types of input a word receives that determine the serial order of the word's phonemes. In one type of input, each word has a tag for each phoneme and each phoneme has nodes. In the second type of input, a context-timing signal feeds information to the word that denotes the correct order of phonemes. To produce the correct order of the phonemes that can be matched to a lexeme, the nodes and the signal must be in sync. The connections between the nodes and the signal via the tag have two types of weights: fast weights that lead to a rapid decay of the connections and slow weights that are more durable and allow the connections to be strengthened. Therefore, the loop processes phonemes at different speeds depending on the weight of their nodes. Slow weights are necessary to allow rehearsal of phonemes, which processes them for long enough to put them in the correct order and match them to a lexeme. Slow weights are also necessary to allow enough time to rehearse a word when it is recalled. The exact nature of the interplay of fast and slow weights still needs to be investigated. However, we know that the decay of the connections is necessary to make room for another tag as soon as the word has been processed.

Figure 7 shows a graphic representation of fast and slow weights of a phoneme.

The signal can be out of sync due to noise. Noise occurs when the brain activates too many phonemes at once. This can happen when we try to speak very fast, which means that many words have to be processed at the same time. We assume that the record of a word includes a tag to the phonemes that can be matched to a lexeme. We also assume that phonemic nodes are not part of the record, as phonemes are stored separately and governed by rules. Like the filter in Page and Norris's (1998) model, the signal has to operate independently to fulfill its function. It is not part of the record of the word. Therefore, when the signal has to deal with too much information, the signal randomly tags nodes to process words based on the number of syllables. Depending on their weight, they fall out of rehearsal quickly or are selected, resulting in an incorrect match to the lexeme.

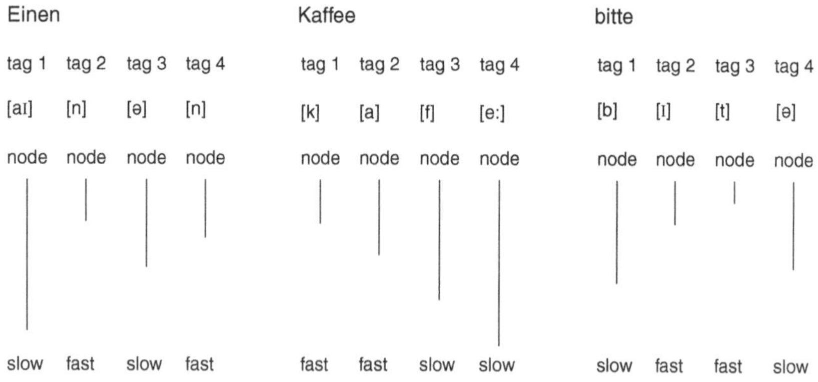

Figure 7. Fast and Slow Weights of Phonemes.

With the context-timing signal that is supposed to put the phonemes in the correct order, we can also explain the phonological similarity effect. If ten words are recalled from a list and they are similar, it is more difficult to recall them on the first attempt than if they are different. When the phonemes are similar, it is naturally more difficult for the signal to discriminate among them in order to determine their correct order. This means that some phonemes are not correctly ordered before the weights decay, and are therefore not processed any further. As a consequence, in this situation we will recall fewer words because, even if the process starts again, this does not change the fact that the phonemes remain similar. The word length effect – longer words are often more difficult to recall than shorter words – can also be explained. It is a matter of weights decaying before all phonemes could be timed by the signal.

All of these details of Page and Norris's (1998) and Burgess and Hitch's (1999) models illustrate how complex the rehearsal process really is when we try to speak. Not only does our brain call up lexemes as well as phonemes, but the subvocal process rehearses these lexemes and phonemes separately as well as together: lexemes are discriminated against other lexemes, phonemes against other phonemes, and tags compete with other tags to try to match them. Nodes go through filters or weights to allow some phonemes more time to be rehearsed than others. A signal influences the order of phonemes. In summary, one phoneme might be at a different stage of rehearsal in the loop than another phoneme and the lexeme might not be ready in Broca's area because the tag is not strong enough. Considering all these different stages of processing, it is quite amazing that in the end the desired combination is matched and the word, which consists of a lexeme and phonemes, can be put into a pre-speech plan – that is, provided the proper morphemes are attached, which in some cases depends on the location of the word in the sentence.

When we make speech errors, we learn from them, so that the next time we say the word we will process the correct combination of the lexeme to its phonemes. Through repeated recall, we improve the record of a word by strengthening and/or adding information. Finally, it needs to be mentioned that the processes of the loop can be impaired in many ways. If there is damage to the left side of the parietal lobe, the trace of a phoneme cannot be prolonged because the temporary store no longer functions, which prevents phoneme sequences to bind and match to a lexeme. If there is damage to the hippocampus (which creates a record of a word), the additional information needed to select the correct phoneme-lexeme combination cannot be called up. If there is damage to the non-mesial region (storage of the record), no lexemes can be recalled. Interestingly, in the case of damage to the non-mesial region, words can still be repeated within a few seconds of being heard, but they cannot be recalled.

5 First and Second Language Acquisition

L1 vs. L2

Every word we know was once new to us. We learn our first words in the first few years of our lives. The way in which we acquire our first words as a child in the language we grow up with (L1) happens under different circumstances than when we learn words in another language (L2) as an adult. However, in each case working memory functions in the same way: it springs into action when needed. Several neurons fire simultaneously, the relevant brain regions and circuits activate, the mechanisms to process a word are set in motion and transmit the information in a fluid and dynamic matter. Attention is directed to an incoming word that is processed in the phonological loop as well as Wernicke's area to eventually create a record in the hippocampus. The workings of working memory are temporary.

If everything goes well, we speak at a rate of two words per second. However, when we speak in our first language as opposed to in another language there are often differences in terms of fluency, accuracy, and complexity of speech (Skehan, 1998; Skehan and Foster, 1997). In general, in first language acquisition, the process of identifying phonemes, lexemes, and establishing a form-to-meaning relationship via a lemma becomes largely automatic, while the first few thousands words are learned around the age of three. A native speaker has the full repertoire of phonemes at his or her disposal although s/he has to learn how phonemes are grouped in syllables, some of which have regular, and some unusual, patterns. A large number of concepts need to be developed in order to identify the lemma. The rules of morphology to grammatically code a word are learned as early as age three and should be automatic by the age of six to eight. Over time, we not only acquire many words but also many meanings of the same word. In second language acquisition, the fluency, accuracy, and complexity of speech depend on the phase of development the person learning that language is in (in the literature this is sometimes referred to as the age of acquisition). We will go into more detail below. In addition to the phase of development, the situation in which the word is acquired also contributes; for example, if the word is encountered in an environment where the learned language is predominantly spoken. Individual factors such as the type of motivation or the background of the speaker also play a role. Finally, successful acquisition depends on the word itself, as there are differences between words in terms of length, similarity, or emotional connotation.

In adult second language acquisition, which reflects the situation of first-year college or university students who learn a language such as German, French, or Spanish, transfer of lexemes with their lemmas and morphological markers takes place from the L1 to the L2. All the factors mentioned – phase of development, learning situation and environment, motivation, background, and the word itself – can be linked to the degree of transfer. In addition, the level of proficiency plays a key role. Beginning learners often transfer lemmas from L1 to L2 directly (de Bot, 1992; Jiang, 2000; Kroll and Dijkstra, 2010). For example, the concept of a house is transferred from the learners' experience growing up in a house in North America to the German word for house (which is "Haus"), although a typical German house might look very different. So sometimes the transfer aids processing words in L2 and sometimes it does not. With an increasing level of proficiency, lemmas are accessed in the L2 without the detour via the L1. Furthermore, the learner also develops lemmas that are unique to the L2.

With regard to the morphological markers, there are different types of bound or system morphemes. They are attached at a later phase to the lexeme as it is processed. The rules that underlie the process of these morphological markers – that is, when and where and how they are attached to words – are quite complex, especially since these rules differ among languages. A good example can be found in late system morphemes, such as tense markers. In English, Third Person Singular Present Tense adds an "-s." In German, verbs add an "-e" for 1.P.Sg. Present Tense, an "-st" for 2.P.Sg., a "-t" for 3.P.Sg. and 2.P.Pl. and an "-en" for 1.P.Pl. and 3.P.Pl. At the beginner's level, learners whose L1 is English often forget to add those morphemes in German, because they are not added in English. This is called negative transfer.

In summary, it is clear that in second language acquisition the processes that surround new word acquisition are not automatic for adult learners. At the beginner's level, much rehearsal and matching needs to take place to create a record of the phonemes and lexemes that are encountered for the first time. This makes beginner language learners an interesting group to research. If the process is not automatic, we need to look at the faculties that determine our brain's capacity to actually process new words in L2, in addition to how the brain actually develops this capacity. The development is linked to our L1, since we acquired our first words at a young age, and learned to speak and develop language as a system. The faculties are: memory, cognition, and language.

Memory

We are born with about 100 billion neurons, the most we will ever have. From birth forward, we lose neurons every day, but fortunately we also create new neurons in certain areas of the brain such as the hippocampus. An adult brain has about 85 billion neurons (Herculano-Houzel, 2009). Once we reach our mid-sixties, however, the number of neurons substantially decreases. In general, our brain relies on the work of its synapses to transmit information between neurons. Synapses number in the trillions because they connect neurons in many ways. Synapses can be formed throughout life and connect nerve cells that previously did not have a connection, although a key phase in synapse formation occurs before the age of six. With regard to language, the neuroanatomical circuits that connect the faculties involved when processing words must also be formed before the age of six.

Just like our bodies need physical exercise in order to stay fit, our synapses benefit from cognitive activity. Synapses that are used are strengthened, while those not used become dormant and eventually dissipate. The prefrontal cortex – where Broca's area is located, which includes the rehearsal component of the phonological loop – becomes an especially important site of synapse use between the ages of eight and twenty-four months (Bauer, 2004). In order to create a record of a word, the hippocampus – which sits deep down in the brain, connected to the amygdala – depends on the information fed to it by the synapses. The hippocampus receives information via the enthornial and perirhinal cortices, a process that then allows it to collect sensory information from other brain regions, for example, from the olfactory bulb, the occipital lobe, and the auditory cortex (Gluck and Myers, 2001). Although much of the development of the hippocampus takes place between the ages of two to four or five, its functions do not reach full development until about the age of eight (Richmond and Nelson, 2007). The record of a word is stored in the non-mesial region, which is adjacent to the hippocampus, although the hippocampus may assist in the retrieval of information. This is why children rarely have memories before ages four or five. If they do, those are very likely to be rekindled images rather than recollections of actual situations or events, unless the memory follows a highly emotional or traumatic event, in which case the release of large amounts of the neurotransmitters serotonin or dopamine or acetylcholine would lead the brain to record and store the salient information. Memory recall is linked to speech; that is, to talking about those memories. In order to talk about memories, the child needs language skills and vocabulary. It is around the age of two and a half that children start to learn more and more words. This in turn contributes to the development of the hippocampus in a process that simply takes time.

Genetics determines the underlying grid of where synaptic connections form, and the way in which these connections function depends on the input of information. Information input is linked to the environment in which a learner is raised. This is particularly important for children, since a rich lexical environment that exposes a child to many words, multiple word meanings, and a variety of word interplay is necessary for the child to acquire a good vocabulary. The brain faculties responsible for language processes and the acquisition of new words have a limited capacity and can only handle a certain amount of information at a time; therefore, the acquisition of new words must be timed and spread apart by spacing them. When we interact with a child, it is important to repeat words, in particular if the words occur in different situations and have a different meaning in each of those situations. To help develop a child's memory, we can read to the child, as s/he will start to remember the story after they heard it several times. However, it is also important to not read the same story three times in a row, but to read it to them every other day or every few days, in order to give the developing brain a chance to process the information. On the alternate days, you may read a different story to the child.

Our memory develops as we grow. According to some psychologists, we form most of our memories between the ages of sixteen to twenty-five. This is called the "reminiscence bump" (Draaisma, 2004). Concurrently, the phonological loop is refined during this time in our life. Of course we also form memories after our mid-twenties, but they are often tied to very emotional events, such as a wedding or car accident. We return to this in Chapter 8, "Word Analysis."

In the previous chapter, we learned that every word has a memory trace that lasts for about half a second but can be prolonged through the mechanisms of the phonological loop. A reliable method with which to measure memory capacity is a memory span test that indicates how many words a person can remember in the correct order. In a typical experiment, a child must listen to a list of ten words and then repeat them in free recall. Pickering and Gathercole (2001) showed that children at the age of four usually remember two words in a row, and at age fifteen they remember four words, if tested on short-term gains. If a similar test uses numbers instead of words, the experiment is called a digit span test. At the age of four, children are able to repeat three numbers and, at the age of fifteen, six.

Two factors play a role when it comes to how the memory span improves. First, around age six the subvocal rehearsal process in the phonological loop starts to develop within the human brain. This rehearsal process is necessary to deal with several items (words/digits) at a time. The second factor involves speed. The faster the loop processes a word, the more words it can process. This requires the refinement of the rehearsal process in combination with the temporary storage of the phonological loop. It is not until the mid-twenties that rehearsal and temporary storage will work at its optimal peak. The reason why children are able to recall more numbers than words in short-term gains is that numbers do not have a rich lexeme that has to be matched to its phonemes. The processing of numbers depends solely on the rehearsal and temporary storage within the loop. If the test is carried out right after the numbers are read to the children, then the numbers are still present. If the test is carried out later, the child will no longer be able to recall the numbers. On a test of long-term memory, children will recall more words than numbers.

Finally, we need to consider the cognitive ability to process and store information. In the 1920s, Swiss psychologist Jean Piaget studied children and developed the theory of cognitive development (Piaget, 1955, 1962). He proposed four stages in the development of a child, in which the last two are related to language. The third stage is called the "concrete operational stage," which starts around age seven and goes until about age eleven. In this stage, the life of a child becomes more structured and therefore memories are more organized and easier to retrieve. The fourth and last stage in a child's development he calls the "formal operational stage." It starts as early as age eleven (although it varies, as for many children it starts age twelve or thirteen) and allows the child to think logically and to solve problems that are increasingly complex. This is also referred to as abstract thinking. It should be noted that these skills need years to develop and are still refined in a person's late teen years (age seventeen or eighteen).

With regard to cognition, we also have to consider the executive control that directs attention to incoming words (Baddeley, 2007) and, as some researchers argue, can keep words that are not immediately processed in a holding pattern (Cowan, 1999). It is located in the prefrontal cortex of the brain. Directing, dividing, and switching attention places a high demand on the cognitive resources. Naturally, it takes time to develop this ability. In a study with children aged three and a half to seven, Diamond and Taylor (1996) used a tapping task that required children to remember two rules as well as to control a natural response: when the experimenter tapped twice with a wooden dowel, the child had to tap once, and vice versa (when the experiment tapped twice, the child had to tap once). The natural response would be for the child to tap as many times as the experimenter did. The study showed that older children were faster and more accurate than younger children, particularly when six years or older. These findings suggest that the prefrontal cortex is functioning well in children around the age of six and up. Further studies have shown that the development of the prefrontal cortex continues until late adolescence to refine the ability of directing, dividing, and switching attention (Davidson et al., 2006; Diamond, 2002; Rothbart and Posner, 2005).

Language

The functions of neurotransmitters – such as serotonin or dopamine or acetylcholine, as well as hormones, proteins, and enzymes that all contribute to the modification or creation of synapses – change over a lifetime and therefore influence language development. Our body and brain develop over time, and five sensitive phases mark the development of our language acquisition:

1. building connections (until 1/until 6 to 8/lifelong)
2. developing strategies (around 8)
3. analyzing abstractions (11 to 14)
4. developing the loop (6 to 16)
5. creating memories (6 to 25/lifelong).

Before we discuss L2 in more detail, we need to know a few things about language development in L1. There are three factors we have to look at in terms of language development:

- vocabulary
- grammar
- strategies.

Between nine and thirteen months a child has the 100 phonemes or so of all the languages in the world at its disposal. It can actually distinguish all those sounds. However, the child adapts to the sounds it hears the most by discriminating phonemes to catalogue the L1 phoneme inventory. Just past one year of age, the child can only distinguish between the phonemes of the language or languages with which it is surrounded. Between four and eight months, children try to say their first sounds, in particular vowels. As Szagun (1996) explains, some children will internally rehearse the sounds they hear, while some will actually try to say them out loud. These sounds are based on an imitation of what the child hears most often, and the sounds are also infused with meaning, for example: Mom-mom-mom-mom.

The first words are spoken out loud, usually around the first birthday. Initially, there are only a few words and they might be mispronounced. However, between eighteen months and two years of age, the so-called vocabulary explosion begins. Now children learn words at a rapid speed, building connections between phonemes and lexemes, and can acquire up to ten new words each day. Initially they make many mistakes: everything that moves is called a "car," and every bird is a "duck" (Clark, 1973). They classify things by shape and need time to discover differences in size, texture, and detail. They start to build a network of words. It is important for them to begin to realize that things and activities have names. For anatomical reasons, the vowel "u" might still cause them trouble to pronounce, as well as the "s." The position of the tongue and the larynx still moves around, until they both find their final position around age six to eight. Vowel-consonant combinations such as "tz" are also challenging. Words that are acquired and spoken are usually short and consist of one or two syllables. At this age, longer words require much effort to imitate and pronounce, although some children will be able to do so with success. In general, somewhere between the age of one and a half to two and a half, most children know about 500 words (Gleason, 2001).

Most of those 500 words are nouns, and many such nouns refer to objects, while some refer to emotional states. Some children will actually combine a noun with a pronoun, such as "I Mom" (probably trying to say: "I want Mommy"), or "I sleep," trying out the first verbs. Even before they can form sentences, children are able to express relations between objects, states, and events with the use of prepositions such as "in" or "under" or "on." Age three to five is a very interesting age in language development, because on the one hand children still imitate their surroundings, while on the other they start to learn the first rules, such as "Nouns get an '-s' in the plural" and "Verbs in 3.P.Sg. get an '-s'." However, it is one thing to learn the rules, but another to know the exception to the rule. So for the next two years, starting at age three, children have to puzzle out morphemes (bound or system morphemes alike) to avoid overextensions. For example, they learn that the simple past ending is "-ed": "she walks" becomes "she walked." So they say things such as "she sleeped," even though a few months before they may have correctly said, "she slept." At that time, they were imitating. At this point, the rules are overextended. Similarly, the plural "mice' – said correctly at the age of three – becomes "mouses" six months later. However, around the age of five children usually solve these mistakes and return to "she slept" and "mice."

At the ages of three to four, sentences become more complex (Tager-Flusberg, 2001). Around this time children are able to say four- or five-word sentences and thereby make meaningful relations between words. They ask questions such as, "Why?" and "Can I play with … ?" Thus, they are able to reverse word order (statement: "I can play with … "). They start to count. At the age of five, their speaking abilities are amazing, although they still have to learn how to apply rules and exceptions, and they will require the next couple of years for practice. Between the ages of six and eight, a child knows about 14,000 words, is able to pronounce those words correctly, can rhyme, and can understand that a word consists of different syllables. These skills are necessary to begin the adventure of learning how to read and write. Although language skills such as reading, writing, listening, and speaking will develop throughout the years, it is believed that if children do not have those abilities between the ages of six and eight, they will never catch up. Initially it was proposed that children need to have those abilities developed by the age of five (Lenneberg, 1967) but this was later extended to six to eight years by researchers such as Korte (2009), who took into account the importance of memory in language development, in particular the circuits set in motion when we process language.

The ability to read and write enables children to make relations between words that are more complex. They learn more about word order (called syntax) and tense markers (for example, passive voice) that become more and more automatic. At the age of eight to ten they also learn that a similar meaning can be expressed using a variety of words and they begin to develop strategies. Eventually, they are able to tell complex stories in a structured way that saves the highlight of the story for last. There are many discussions as to how to classify strategies. For language learning, Oxford (1990) developed a practical system. Oxford distinguishes between six categories:

- cognitive strategies (for example, analyzing a problem by using prior knowledge and to infer the solution)
- metacognitive strategies (for example, planning ahead or self-monitoring one's speech)
- memory strategies (reviewing/repeating and verifying and creating associations)
- affective strategies (for example, encouraging oneself)
- social strategies (for example, asking questions)
- compensation strategies (for example, guessing).

When learning a new word, memory strategies are a key component. To review and verify describes the process of rehearsing phonemes and matching them to a lexeme well. Repeated rehearsal is necessary in order to facilitate a successful lexeme match and to create a record that will be stored and later recalled from long-term memory. Associations may assist identifying lexemes if the new word reminds us of another word we know already. However, associations may also create problems. If a learner attempts to acquire too many new words at a time by creating associations – for example, via a word field or word tree – it will overburden the cognitive load. This presents a particular issue if those words are phonologically similar, because the loop will require extra time and effort to distinguish between them.

Studies have shown that children use the lexemes and phonemes of words they already know in order to process new words. In a study carried out with twelve-year-old children who spoke Cantonese as their first language and who began to learn English in Hong Kong at the age of three or four, Cheung (1996) used two syllable non-words and asked children to repeat them back. We have to keep in mind that a test of non-words only measures the ability to rehearse phonemes. Cheung compared the children's scores from the non-word test to their scores on an earlier vocabulary test that measured the children's ability to learn new words in English. Results showed that children with low scores on the test that measured their ability to learn new words also scored low on the test that asked them to repeat non-words. This confirms other studies in this area that demonstrate the positive influence of the ability to repeat non-words on vocabulary development (Gathercole and Baddeley, 1989; Service, 1992). However, some of the children in Cheung's study who did well learning new words did not do well when asked to repeat non-words. How did they achieve such high scores on new words if they could not process the phonemes of the new words with success? A possible explanation may be that, starting to learn English at the age of three or four, these children had already acquired a good repertoire of phonemes and lexemes of English words by the age of twelve, and they inferred that knowledge to the new words.

A study from French and O'Brien (2008) reached the same conclusion. They carried out a study with eleven-year-old French students in Quebec who were learning English, to determine if non-word repetition impacts the learning of grammar and vocabulary in a five-month intensive English course. They did find that the ability to rehearse non-words positively influenced the learning of grammar but had little effect on vocabulary. Similar to Cheung's study, this result seems to contradict what we would expect. However, most of the children had been exposed to English before and in fact had a good knowledge of many English words. Although French and O'Brien's study is difficult to assess, because many things can happen over a time period of five months that can influence a child's ability to learn, it does strengthen the view that children who are eight years or older use knowledge of words they have already acquired in order to learn new words.

Around age eleven or twelve, things change again when learning a language. As described above, the growing body undergoes physical changes and also alters chemicals in the bloodstream. This affects the brain. New synapses form that enable the youth to think logically, to solve problems, and to understand abstract relations. The psychologist Hasselhorn (2005) describes how children or youth at this age start to use abstract words such as "Freiheit" [freedom]. Some abstract words such as "love" have been used before, as early as three years of age, but at that time they were used in a direct relation as a concrete noun and by imitation ("I love Mommy."). Now children or youth develop metacognitive skills and use those skills to become aware of how language is used; that is, they begin to understand how language works as a system.

In general, children need time to develop the capacity to process words. Not only is the hippocampus not fully up and running until about eight years of age, but the phonological loop – the rehearsal as well as the temporary store – also develops throughout the years. The rehearsal and the temporary store of the loop begin to develop at birth, and by the age of six they function well; however, the interplay between the two still needs to be refined (Gathercole et al., 2004). The subvocal rehearsal processes in particular become more efficient over time and are completely refined by age six to sixteen. In addition, the loop must interact with Wernicke's and Broca's area as well as the hippocampus, a process that needs time and practice to be optimized. The capacity to process words is at its peak in the mid-twenties (Korte, 2009).

It should also be pointed out, as it was by Nagy (1997), that the vocabulary explosion in children, which starts around age two, does not stop when we reach age sixteen. We continue to learn words and create memories throughout life. Naturally language/vocabulary proficiency is also linked to the kind of education one receives as a child, a youth, and a young adult. Carrying on with that education after high school, for example, by enrollment in trade school or college, the vocabulary will continue to grow exponentially until the mid-twenties. However, it must be noted that to provide the circumstances for input – that is, to provide a situation in which we will encounter new words – is one thing. But having the ability to process all those words is another. Therefore, the development of the phonological loop should not be underestimated. It should also be noted that, just as the interplay of the phonological loop with other language and memory faculties is perfected between the ages of sixteen and twenty-five, this time frame is concurrent with the stage that some psychologists (Draaisma, 2004) view as the age in which we form most of our memories.

Coming back to those five phases – building connections; developing strategies; analyzing abstractions; developing the loop; creating memories – the question is what happens when we learn another language. Naturally, someone who is exposed to that language during one of the phases will have an advantage, as s/he interacts with the language during a sensitive phase. Someone who is exposed to another language during all of the phases should become bilingual. Of course, this will depend on that person's will to learn. It takes effort to learn a language, with its new words and grammar, and in order to be successful we must practice – we must write and speak in the new language. Our success also depends on the environment in which the language is acquired, in particular if the learned language is predominantly spoken in that environment. Being immersed in the L2 environment fosters language development, as it provides increased exposure to both literal and contextual aspects of the language. It also gives the learner an opportunity to talk to a native speaker, and thereby provides greater opportunities for communication, which is one of the key motivations for learning a language. We will go into more detail in Chapter 9, "Learning and Teaching."

Missing one of the five phases in the development of our language acquisition may affect the fluency, accuracy, or complexity of speech. This applies to vocabulary as well as to grammar. The great amount of input we receive as we learn our L1, compared to an L2, is often underestimated. Researchers generally agree that it is best to start to learn another language before the age of eleven. However, it is equally important to continue to learn and practice the L2 beyond that age, as pointed out by Singleton (1995, 2007; Cook and Singleton, 2014), who carried out much work in this area.

A good example can be seen in French Immersion programs in Canada, where children in elementary school (age five to eleven) who speak a different L1 than French (L2) at home are taught in French. If these children do not continue to learn and speak French in middle school (age eleven to fourteen) or high school (age eleven or fourteen to eighteen), they will forget much of their written and spoken French by the time they go to college or university. On the plus side, it is possible to still become bilingual when learning another language for the first time at college or university. From my experience as a teacher of German as a foreign language in North America, I do have students who had no previous experience with any language apart from English. They start with first-year German at the age of eighteen, and within two years some of them write and speak German fluently and master the language well. Those who spend some time in Germany during their studies become especially proficient.

To learn another language after our mid-twenties will be more difficult, but it is still possible, in particular with intrinsic motivation. Among other things, intrinsic motivation is fostered by interpersonal relatedness, which means to be engaged in the process of learning for personal reasons (Deci and Ryan, 1985, 2002). For example, if we learn another language because a friend or loved one speaks that language, we can become proficient even if we start to learn the language after those sensitive phases during the first twenty-five years of our lives.

In summary, the potential to form new synapses is determined by genetics. The way in which the child, youth, or young adult makes use of that potential is influenced by the input s/he receives. The process of phoneme and lexeme rehearsal needs to be developed and refined over time. Children go through a vocabulary explosion starting around the age of two, but more importantly they must understand concepts of lexemes and multiple meanings, including abstractions, that develop around eleven or twelve years of age. We also need to remember that the grammatical coding of words, in particular bound or system morpheme attachment, has a delayed start, since naturally a child must first acquire a sufficient number of words before the child can code words with proper grammar, such as "I sleep, she sleeps, we sleep." The age of three to five is particularly interesting. Once some of the rules have been acquired, though, new words, including their potential system and bound morphemes, integrate smoothly into the child's vocabulary. It is worthwhile to ask how the grammatical coding works when we acquire new words in another language, since morphemes are language-specific.

This is something we will discuss in the next chapter. The process of word acquisition is lifelong, although the capacity to do so is at its peak in the mid-twenties. Overall, language learning goes through five developmental phases that happen naturally as we mature. If we miss one or more of those phases, it will be more difficult, but not impossible, to learn another language. Much of our success depends on the underlying processes of acquiring words; that is, how much our cognitive load can handle. The core processes are the same in L1 and L2. If we acquire an L2 at the same time we acquire an L1, we should speak both languages with fluency, accuracy, and with a high degree of complexity. If we acquire an L2 later in life, we can use our knowledge of the L1. Depending on other factors such as the environment in which we acquire the language, as well as our proficiency level and motivation, this can have a positive or negative effect on our L2 acquisition. This will be the topic of Chapter 6, "The Bilingual Lexicon and Speaker."

A Word on Pronunciation

In addition to vocabulary, grammar, and strategies, we must also discuss how the speaker pronounces a word correctly. It is a challenge for the child's young brain to discriminate phonemes and match them to lexemes. Around the ages of two or three, parents will hear all kinds of words from their children. A good example is the pronunciation of "bathtub." It is possible the child may replace a similar type phoneme such as "p" for "b," as they are both bilabial plosives: "pathtub." Other possibilities occur in the use of a very different phoneme, as it seems easier to pronounce in that particular combination of phonemes, such as "m" (bilabial nasal) for "t" (alveolar plosive) – "bathmup" – or replacing part of the word with one that has been heard before, such as "mug" for "tub" – "bathmug" – or to leave out a phoneme, such as the "t" – "bathub." Some children have difficulties with the "th" and might say "baftub." In German, some children have difficulties with "s."

The mistakes occur because children acquire the first few thousand words aurally. They listen to the sounds of words. Because they do not yet know how to read, they cannot match a sound to a letter or a phoneme to a grapheme or graphemes. They will learn how to read much later, around the age of five or six. Instead, they have to puzzle out the sounds of words, a task that can present quite a challenge. If a child demonstrates a persistent pronunciation problem, a speech therapist can help the child to utter those sounds correctly. If these pronunciation problems are not treated in time, they can cause more problems later on, for example, in the incorrect use of morphemes, since the pronunciation of morphemes needs to be accurate in order to grammatically encode a word. Therefore, problems with hearing or speaking can affect the development of grammar, and a small pronunciation problem that could have been corrected by a speech therapist early on in a child's life may progress to a language impairment if not treated in time.

Eventually, most children decipher how to pronounce all of the phonemes. As Doughty (2003) explains, when children acquire their first language, they learn phonemes with prosody (stress, rhythm, intonation) and coarticulation (vowels that overlap and/or consonants pronounced in close succession). In the first year of their development, children rehearse phonemes and use rehearsal to discriminate the phonemes of their first language from the phonemes of other languages. Prosody and coarticulation help children to discriminate between which phonemes they actually need. After about thirteen months, phonemes that were not rehearsed dissipate. Therefore, when acquiring another language, usually the challenge of pronouncing words correctly begins again, because the phonemes of other languages are no longer readily available – unless the language learner had sufficient input from two languages during the first year of life and continued to receive such input throughout childhood, in which case the pronunciation in both languages should be perfect, because Wernicke's area has catalogued two phoneme inventories: one for L1 and one for L2.

The physical parts involved in pronunciation, such as the tongue, lips, and larynx, continue to develop and change when we are younger. Therefore, it is easier for a younger learner to acquire the pronunciation of the phonemes of another language past thirteen months than it is for an adult learner.

Most of us need to practice the phonemes of a new language in order to pronounce them properly. However, the language itself is also a factor. Mistakes made by adult learners of another language include using incorrect stress, intonation, rhythm, or syllabification. English and German, for example, use a pronunciation system that is primarily based on stress, and less so on syllables. If a native German speaker speaks English, we will usually be able to detect an accent, especially when the speaker pronounces vowels or consonants; however, the prosody and coarticulation are correct for the most part. Some other languages are more difficult. French, for example, places more emphasis on syllabification than English or German; therefore, native English or German speakers who wish to learn French may find it a challenge not only to master the French manner of speech, but also to use the correct coarticulation when they pronounce French words. Likewise, French native speakers are sometimes difficult to understand when they speak English, because their prosody and coarticulation are different.

When we begin to learn a new language past the age of eleven to fourteen, it becomes very likely that we will carry our native accent into the new language. There are some exceptions to this. Someone who has a refined ear, such as a musician, may be able to distinguish subtleties in sound and intonation well enough to achieve credible pronunciation in the learned language. This is more likely to occur if the learner begins to speak the new language more often than his or her native language, especially if s/he is immersed in the new language environment. In a study of native Polish speakers who lived in Germany, Molnár (2010) showed that the degree to which a person speaks with an accent depends not only on the individual learner and his or her background, but also on the learning situation.

In a series of experiments, Archibald and Gathercole (2006) highlighted the role of prosody and coarticulation in the process of phoneme acquisition. We know that the ability to repeat non-words (to rehearse phonemes), in combination with accessing words that have been acquired already (to rehearse lexemes), is a key factor in learning new words. Archibald and Gathercole showed that children with SLI not only have problems with non-words but also find it difficult to repeat words in the correct order; that is, the order they were presented to them. Twenty children had to do three free recall tasks with the use of digits, non-words, and words. Fourteen children performed poorly on the digit and word task, but all of them performed poorly on non-words. The difference between non-words and words is that non-words do not have a lexeme that can be easily identified. However, digits cannot be easily identified either, and yet these children performed better on the digit task compared to the non-word task. Testing digits is a good indicator of the function of the phonological loop because, similar to non-words, digits do not have a rich lexeme and their processing depends on the interplay between rehearsal and temporary storage. However, as Archibald and Gathercole point out, in order to process the phonemes of the non-words, we do not rely exclusively on the phonological loop. The child may not immediately recognize the non-word as such and may try to find a lexeme (with the assistance of the Wernicke's area, as well as the hippocampus) in order to identify the phonemes. This search process uses up time that is lost when no lexeme is found and the memory trace vanishes. If the child thinks that the non-word may in fact be a word, s/he may also try to look for prosodic cues. However, neither of those two processes of inquiry occur when the child handles a number, because a number is easily identified as such. In order to find out more about the role played by prosody and coarticulation, Archibald and Gathercole (2007) carried out another study, this time with children without SLI. They investigated the phoneme at the phoneme level. Archibald and Gathercole created twenty-four syllables of different combinations of consonants and vowels. They tested twenty-six children in two groups (group 1: nine- to thirteen-year-olds; group 2: five- to eight-year-olds). In the first test, the children heard a non-word made up of three to five of those twenty-four syllables. They were asked to repeat it immediately. In the second test, children heard a sequence of three to five of the twenty-four syllables in a row, each pronounced separately, to indicate that they did not make up a non-word, and were asked to repeat back the order of the sequence. Results showed that children performed better on the first test than on the second: they demonstrated greater accuracy when they repeated non-words than when they were asked to recall the sequence of the syllables. In the non-word repetition, children made fewer mistakes when they recalled the vowels compared to the consonants. This is because consonants change in syllables, whereas vowels usually do not. For example, three syllables were "ba," "ta," and "da." Naturally, it is more difficult to remember the consonants, as there is a different consonant before the same vowel. It is likely that children recalled non-words with greater accuracy than sequences of syllables because the syllables of non-words connect through prosody and coarticulation, whereas isolated sequences of syllables do not.

We have now discussed the factors involved when we learn another language in terms of memory, cognitive ability, and language skills. In most cases, to learn another language means to learn a second language after a first language has been acquired. However, it is possible to acquire two (or more) languages simultaneously. In fact, children can learn up to four languages at the same time as long as they have a need to do so (Korte, 2009). For example, if the mother speaks German, and the father speaks French, but the family lives in England, where the child attends an English-speaking school and has a best friend who is from Spain, then the child has reason to learn all of these languages. Such cases may be rare, but today more and more children grow up bilingual, trilingual, or even polylingual; that is, they learn more than two languages at the same time. In most cases, however, a child will favor one of the languages. This type of bilingualism is an excellent source from which to investigate how words of different languages interact in our minds or, more precisely, how we process phonemes and lexemes of different languages when we first encounter them, as well as once we recall them from long-term memory. This is the topic of the following chapter.

6 The Bilingual Lexicon and Speaker

Vocabulary

Most Germanic languages have more than 100,000 words, and that number continues to grow as new words are created every year. Most of us only know half this number of words because the other half consists of specialized vocabulary. In daily communication we hardly use 10 percent of those 50,000 words. When we learn another language, we need to absorb thousands of new words. Knowing about 5,000 words will allow most people to communicate in most situations (Schmitt, 2010b).

In Chapter 5, "First and Second Language Acquisition," we learned that children form semantic networks growing up; that is, they build a network of words that are connected via their lemma and/or lexeme. A semantic network is a product. A question we should ask with regard to second language acquisition is whether we process a new word in L2 via the same circuits with which we process a word in L1. Another question is whether L1 and L2 share the same semantic network.

It is important to distinguish a semantic network from the overall language network.

In Chapter 3, "Synaptic Connections," we learned that this language network consists of neuroanatomical circuits formed through the hardware within the phonological loop, Broca's and Wernicke's area, the hippocampus, amygdala, and several cortices. In that scenario, a network describes a process.

The main question pursued in this book is what actually happens when we encounter, and subsequently try to process, a word in another language. Naturally, some of the phonemes in different languages – for example, German and English – sound very different. In some languages – for example, Japanese – they are entirely different. What about the lexeme? In the speaker's first language, each word is associated with a concept, which is best defined as a mental image that corresponds to the word. The concept is expressed through the lemma of the lexeme. One of the questions is whether we learn a new word in a new language together with a new concept, or whether the new word borrows a familiar concept from a word we already know in the L1.

In language acquisition, the process of matching a word with a concept is at the heart of how we learn and remember, and also how we sometimes fail to remember, that is, how we forget. These processes apply to our first and second languages alike. To make a concept-word match is somewhat like playing a game of tennis. Sometimes you hit an ace; that is, the word matches a concept one-for-one. Sometimes you hit the ball outside; that is, you cannot possibly find a match. Most often, however, the ball is played back and forth, one of those endless rallies where, by the end, you are so exhausted you wonder why you even started it. A similar procedure happens in the brain when we encounter a word we have not seen or heard before. In order to understand the new word, the brain must find a concept that connects the new word to its existing reference system, also known as our world. So how does a concept fit with a lexeme? In Chapter 1, "A New Word," we learned that a lexeme is an abstract unit that describes the form-to-meaning relationship of a single word. It consists of a lemma and a morphological marker. The concept is matched onto a lexeme via the lemma. It is necessary to have the lemma as a mediator within the lexeme because, on the one hand, a concept that is expressed through the lexeme can be difficult to define and, on the other hand, there can be several ways to grammatically code a concept, and some of those ways may in turn change the concept. Morphemes help to create the grammatical code, and the lexeme contains information in its morphological markers as to what possible morphemes might be encoded.

Much research has been carried out to investigate whether or not words of two different languages are stored in the same lexicon in the non-mesial region. Over the years researchers have proposed many models that attempt to depict what the bilingual lexicon looks like and how words are selected in the brain of the bilingual speaker (for example, the models by de Bot, 1992, 2004; De Groot, 1992; Dijkstra and Van Heuven, 1998, 2002; Kroll and Stewart, 1994 [new version Kroll et al., 2002]). These models were developed in the Netherlands and are based on studies with adult second language learners (Dutch: L1, English: L2). These researchers generally agree that more than one language can be processed at the same time and words in different languages can be accessed simultaneously. Most importantly, the lemma of the L1 and the lemma of the L2 can be linked. When speaking an L2, a speaker can access a concept via the L1 or directly from the L2. However, the degree to which concepts are shared and accessed by L1 and L2 is a question that has not yet been answered.

Most researchers assume that there is a conceptual overlap between L1 and L2 for some words and not for others. Regarding this issue, Pavlenko (2009) developed a scale that ranges from conceptual equivalence to near equivalence to partial non-equivalence and finally to non-equivalence. The advantage of such a scale is that it takes into account subtle differences between concepts such as "der Kaffee" and "the coffee." Most researchers will agree that both languages, L1 and L2, are active when we recall a word, and that the selection of phonemes and lexemes is not tied to one language. When we look for a word, lexemes and phonemes activate within our brain, and we then need to discriminate between them. These can be lexemes and phonemes from two languages. The most activated combination of lexemes and phonemes is then the one that our brain selects as correct.

Some researchers (for an overview, see Kroll and Dijkstra, 2010) have discussed whether there is a language tag in word recall and, if so, at what part of the process this language tag would come into play. The function of a language tag would be to only allow the activation of lexemes in one language and deactivate words in the other language. The real question, though, is whether a language tag is necessary. Phonemes, lexemes, and morphemes exchange information with one another as the brain processes them. Each of them contains information that is language-specific. Depending on the language, some or all phonemes are language-specific, which means they can only be used in that language in conjunction with their integral information. For example, if you learn the vowel "a" in German, you will see that it is pronounced by gathering air in the back of your mouth rather than in the front, such as English "a." Other phonemes in German are identical to English; however, these are processed with tags that determine serial order; therefore the appropriate syllables align during the process. Again, an extra language tag seems unnecessary. In the case of lexemes, the process is more complicated. Each lexeme has a lemma that expresses the concept of the word. A lemma can be language-specific but it can also be shared. A speaker of lower proficiency usually borrows the L1 concept to express the L2 word in order to be efficient. In this case, the learner will often make compromises to get his or her message across. A higher-proficiency speaker can modify the concept according to the needs of the L2 word. In some cases where no equivalent exists in the L1, the speaker can develop and acknowledge a new concept, which means that the L2 word gets its own lemma. So, while some lemmas are accessed via L1, others are accessed directly in L2. Each lexeme also has a morphological marker to indicate where a potential bound or system morpheme can be attached, if necessary. Those morphemes are language-specific as well. As explained, there are different types of morphemes. Early system morphemes occur at the lemma level; for example, the plural "-s" as the lemma will match a concept expressing two or more of something and not just one. Late system morphemes attach at the grammar level, for example Third Person Singular Present Tense "-s." The verb recalled – for example, "walk" – is always the same, as one merely attaches the "-s." Lastly, bridge system morphemes are marked at the lemma level but put into form at the grammar level – for example, the possessive "-s." In other languages, these morphemes are different. German has many ways of forming the plural, which includes "-e," "-en," "-er," and "-s" endings. In addition, some nouns change their vowels. In regards to verb conjugation, verbs add an "-e" for 1. Person Singular Present Tense, an "-st" for 2.P.Sg., a "-t" for 3.P.Sg. and 2.P.Pl. and an "-en" for 1. and 3.P.Pl., and in addition some verbs change their vowels in 2. and 3.P.Sg.

In summary, it can be argued that a language tag would speed up the rehearsal process, in particular when selecting the correct morpheme. On the other hand, the exchange of information between phonemes, lexemes, and morphemes seems to be rich, with enough language specificity to make the existence of a language tag redundant.

Were a language tag to speed up the selection of morphemes, how much of a difference would that make in the overall process from recall to the pre-speech plan? To answer that question, we need to analyze whether this process takes more time in L2 than in L1. Naturally, when we begin to learn another language there are many words we do not know, so we find ourselves in a situation where, although we want to say something, we do not have the words to express ourselves. Or we start a sentence, realize that we do not know the word we are looking for, and have to either adjust the sentence or substitute another word. In this case, we apply strategies as we guess or infer the meaning of the words we have used. In other cases, we may start a new sentence altogether, or ask for help. These maneuvers take more time, which reduces the speed with which we can communicate. However, we should note that most of those situations above occur in speakers with a lower level of proficiency. Of course, speakers with a high level of proficiency are also lost for words at times, but no more so than the average native speaker. Returning to our earlier question as to how the actual process of word recall in L2 compares to that of L1, we have to distinguish between three phases: the initial call-up, the discrimination process, and the grammatical encoding of the word.

The initial call-up is an identical process in both L1 and L2, because of the way Broca's area brings records and phonemes of both languages forward at the same time, if needed. To recall a word from memory in order to use and speak it depends much on the rehearsal of phonemes and a successful lexeme match. Some lemmas are accessed directly in the L2, others via the L1. In either case, lexemes from both languages are brought up when we try to recall a word. The lexeme activated the most, and matched with its phonemes, is the one selected and put into a pre-speech plan. If Broca's area approves the plan, we pronounce the word, in either our L1 or L2.

The speed of the discrimination process depends on the speaker's level of proficiency, as a speaker with low proficiency will often use the lemma of the L1 to express a word in L2. The transfer might take a few more milliseconds than accessing a word directly in L2, as a highly proficient speaker most likely would do. When lemmas are shared, the amount of time needed for the transfer is minimal, though. Hesitation often occurs at an intermediate level of proficiency where a speaker cannot decide which lemma to use. Furthermore, the speaker's level of proficiency has an impact on the accuracy and complexity of the speech. If the speaker is not able to access a lemma directly in the L2, s/he may use a word in the L2 even though s/he does not understand its full meaning. Let's go back to the example of the "Kaffee." If you encounter that word as described at the airport in Hamburg, there is a good chance you will form the lemma of "Kaffee" and not "coffee." However, if you learn via a textbook, in a language course, that the direct German translation of "coffee" is "Kaffee," then you will be likely to form the lemma of "Kaffee" via the lemma of "coffee." You would, in this case, assume they are the same. This is why if you then go to Germany and drink a "Kaffee" for the first time, the size and strength of the "Kaffee" may surprise you. A highly proficient bilingual speaker knows these differences from experience, but a learner at the beginner's level usually does not; that is, unless s/he gained experience when s/he ordered a "Kaffee" in Germany. This is also an indicator of the individual differences between speakers, a factor that should not be underestimated. Some learners are eager, right from the start when they first encounter another language, to absorb everything unique about words in that language, while others prefer to try to compare the words of the other language with the words of their own language.

Finally, when we look at the speed of word processes in L1 and L2, we also need to distinguish between the lexemes and phonemes that form a word vs. the grammatical encoding of that word with a morpheme. This reflects a general distinction between vocabulary and grammar. Before a morpheme can be put into the pre-speech plan, it needs to be attached to a lexeme. During the matching process in Broca's area, the morpheme feeds information back to the lexeme and thereby also to the phonemes and vice versa. In L1, this process is largely automatic once we acquire our L1 as children. In L2 it is not automatic, unless a speaker is highly proficient. Consequently it can take milliseconds more to match the correct morpheme onto the lexeme.

When we consider the overall process – from initial call-up; to rehearsing, discriminating, and matching; to grammatical encoding and final check before pronunciation – a language tag might save some milliseconds when L2 lemmas are accessed via L1 or to attach a morpheme. However, the language tag will need to be activated, which also takes time. Therefore, it might not make that much of a difference. Activating a language tag certainly adds to the complexity of the overall process, which is something our brain attempts to avoid, as it operates on the principle of efficiency. In conclusion, I would therefore argue that a language tag is not necessary.

In summary, the relationship of L1 and L2 words in the lexicon is indeed complex and depends on various factors. Apart from the speaker's level of proficiency and individual motivation, as well as his or her background and the learning environment in which s/he finds him- or herself, which may change over time, we also have to consider the way in which the word category (content vs. function words) and word group (length, similarity, emotion) has an impact on the bilingual lexicon and speaker. This will be explored in Chapter 7, "Word Analysis."

Let's turn back to the second question we asked at the beginning of this chapter. Is the semantic network shared in both L1 and L2? We know that children build semantic networks of words as they learn their L1. Naturally we would like to build such a network in the L2 as well. We know that lemmas can be shared between L1 and L2 and that the acquisition of a lemma in L2 is linked to the proficiency level and individual preferences of the speaker. A speaker with a lower level of proficiency will often access a lemma via the L1, whereas a speaker with a higher level of proficiency can often access the L2 lemma directly, which is precisely how to build a network of words. Another factor is the phase of acquisition the learner is in (see Chapter 5, "First and Second Language Acquisition," with regard to the five phases of language learning). Therefore, as Meara (1984) points out, the nature of the network will vary from speaker to speaker. Although the L1 network also varies from speaker to speaker, the degree of complexity and variation is higher within the L2 network, since links form between L1 words as well as between L1 and L2 words. The degree of variation is particularly high when it comes to examples of words unique to a language. In this case, it would be difficult for the speaker to access the word's concept via the L1. However, despite this additional consideration, we can assume that L1 and L2 share the semantic network to some degree.

Code Switching

Much of the debate on the bilingual lexicon centers on code switching. Research in this area helps us to understand more about lexical and grammatical processes. Code switching describes the phenomenon that occurs when a speaker uses more than one language to express an idea. Sometimes this is done on purpose, but other times this occurs when the speaker has no other choice, because s/he is unable to recall the word s/he wants to say at that moment. There are three types of code switching:

- inter-sentential (from sentence to sentence, or from part of a sentence to another part)
- intra-sentential (from word to word in the same sentence)
- inner-sentential (within the same word).

Code switching can often occur with children between the ages of two and four. For example, I noticed this in the family of some friends of mine, who are native speakers of German but who live in Canada, which means that their children grow up bilingual German and English (German spoken at home, English spoken in kindergarten). During a recent visit, I observed their three-year-old son as he played with a toy screwdriver. He used the word "schraubing," which he must have composed of "schrauben" (to screw, for example, to fasten a screw on a loose board) and the English progressive form "-ing." Most impressive is that German does not have a progressive form, so the boy must have inserted the form to emphasize movement, although in German the lemma of "schrauben" comprises movement. Children who grow up with two languages usually disentangle these types of code switches by the time they are five years old. Code switches are quite common. They indicate the activation of both languages (de Bot and Schreuder, 1993; Green, 1986; Myers-Scotton, 2003). Most code switches occur at the lexeme or phoneme level when the speaker discriminates between phonemes and lexemes of both languages in order to rehearse and match them for speaking. Therefore, since the word is prepared in both languages, it is possible to speak either, up until the final stages of processing. The example noted above, where the boy of three attached a morpheme of one language to a word in another, is rare. This is because the learner usually attaches morphemes slightly later in the rehearsal process. In this example, the "-ing" form that the boy attached tells us that at three years old, his brain has not fully processed the lemma of "schrauben." If the lemma process were complete, he would not need to emphasize the movement of the verb by adding "-ing," since movement is part of the lemma of the German word. From this example we learn that a child's brain needs some time to mature before it can properly arrange words in the lexicon. This is true for children who grow up with two languages, but also for those who grow up with just the one. Of course, it is more of a challenge for the developing brain to handle two languages at a time, which means that language development may appear to take slightly longer for bilingual children. However, we can expect that, by the age of five, bilingual children will have sorted their language-specific morphemes and will no longer produce mixed words such as "schraubing."

Gergely (2007), who observed her son Jamie from the age two years and six months up to three years as he grew up bilingually in Hungarian and English, found several instances of inner-sentential code switching. In one example Jamie attached a Hungarian past tense marker to an English verb. In another example, this time of an intra-sentential code switch, he avoided English articles but used Hungarian ones instead. These instances of code switching, Gergely explains, were within the rules of English and Hungarian grammar. The Hungarian article replaces the English article in the same position that the English article should preserve the determiner phrase. The Hungarian past tense markers attached to English verbs show the same kind of overgeneralization (when the speaker applies the rule of regular past tense to all verbs, even though some verbs are irregular) that children who learn English as an L1 at that age do.

These examples are examples of processing lexemes and morphemes. They show that children raised with two languages of more or less equal input only use one set of neuroanatomical circuits for both languages. To return to our question about proficiency and/or phases of acquisition related to age. Do children or young adults or adults who learn another language later in life also use only one set of circuits, in the sense that they expand the existing set, or do they develop a new circuit set for the language they are learning? With regard to those who grow up with two languages, the question is always whether or not the input from both languages has been equal. This is not only important with regard to lexemes and morphemes but even more so for phonemes. With regard to phonemes, after about the age of one, a child can only distinguish between the phonemes it hears the most. For a child growing up with one language those are the phonemes of that language; for a child growing up with two languages, those are the phonemes of both languages. If the input is not equal, the phonemes of the language that is less present in the child's environment will take longer to be distinguished. The child will need more time to catalogue those phonemes and reproduce them accurately. With regard to lexemes and morphemes, this is discussed in the next section.

Circuits

We are still asking the first question we raised at the beginning of this chapter. Are words in L1 and L2 processed with the same neuroanatomical circuits that spring into action or not? To process a word we need to take into account all of the information a lexeme has, which in addition to the lemma also includes the morphological marker. The morphological markers are usually language-specific. An actual morpheme is attached at a later stage of the process when the speaker recalls a word. First, the record that includes the lexeme is called up, then the speaker rehearses and matches the phonemes, and then a possible morpheme is attached, and the morpheme feeds information back to the lexemes and phonemes. Therefore, the lexical processes are combined with the grammatical processes. We can then ask whether a separate circuit is used for grammatical processes. Moreover, does someone who speaks another language use the same circuit for lexical processes but not grammatical processes? How much does that depend on the age at which the speaker acquired the L2? We know that speakers who grow up with two languages use one circuit for lexical processes. We have not answered the question as to whether speakers who acquire another language later in life also do that. Finally, we need to ask if that might be related to the level of proficiency. If the speaker does, indeed, make use of two networks, are they both active at the same time?

To answer the above question – whether we use one neuroanatomical circuit or two when we speak a second language – some studies turn to the use of neuroimaging technology. However, we must keep in mind that neuroimages are not always an accurate measure of which brain regions activate as the participant carries out a lexical task. While neuroimages can provide possible insight, many factors contribute to the overall process of successful word acquisition and recall.

One of those studies comes from Kim, who as early as 1997 used fMRI technology to investigate second language acquisition. Kim and his colleagues (Kim et al., 1997) designed a study with two groups of adult participants. The first group of six participants had been exposed to another language since infancy, while the other group of six participants had been exposed to another language between the ages of ten to twelve and later spent an extended amount of time in the country where the second language was predominantly spoken. The participants were almost thirty years of age at the time of the test, and all subjects reported to be using both languages equally. All participants were asked to recall what they had done in either the morning, afternoon, or evening of the previous day. In order to avoid head movement that would distort the imaging, participants had to use "inner speech": they were to say the words in their head but not to pronounce them. As this is an unusual task, it was practiced before the imaging took place. The participants were bilingual in a wide range of languages from English and Turkish, Spanish and English, English and Japanese, to Italian and German. All in all, ten languages were tested. Despite testing different languages with various degrees of similarity, and despite the fact that all subjects reported to be fluent in both languages at the time of testing, and despite that the task had been practiced, those who had first been exposed to the other language as infants seemed to use the same circuit in Broca's area, whereas those who had been exposed after the age of ten used separate circuits in Broca's area.

The question is, what do those circuits represent? A circuit is a combination of neurons and synapses that provides the mechanism to process certain information. We have to keep in mind that the circuit within Broca's area is only one part of the speech process. First the brain must recall the record of the word from the non-mesial region, then it must rehearse the phonemes recalled from Wernicke's area in the phonological loop, then it must either match these phonemes to lexemes successfully or contact the hippocampus for additional information on how the record of the word was created. It is only after all of this that the next phase, which consists of grammatical coding, takes place. System or bound morphemes feed information back to the rehearsal process of lexemes and phonemes before they are attached. This affects the order that words are put in to form a sentence. The monitoring system in speech production can send words back to be rehearsed again if the word does not match the lexeme and/or phonemes that were needed. A good example of this occurs when the speaker makes speech errors. The monitoring system can also send a word back to look for a different one. In Kim's study, we cannot determine how accurate, informative, and error-free the speech was, because participants did not actually speak. We also do not know to what degree the inner speech was monitored. But we do know that proficient bilingual adults had to talk about what they had done the previous day and, for that purpose, they had to recall words silently and grammatically encode and put those words into a sentence. Grammatical errors would be attributed to the grammatical coding; non-fluent speech or odd choice of words or incorrect words would be attributed to the rehearsal and/or matching process that brought up a mix of lexemes and phonemes on which the brain could not completely discriminate in a timely manner.

The rehearsal of the loop and the grammatical coding are both part of the Broca's area, whereas the temporary storage of the loop is located in the parietal lobe. The question is if participants who acquired another language later in life used the second circuit for lexical as well as grammatical processing in that language or only for one of those two components of speech production. We should not forget to note the fact that, in general, our brain operates on the principle of efficiency. Using a second circuit requires much effort and energy. The number of words in a language exceeds more than 100,000. It would be challenging to use a separate network to process words. To process a new word, the loop must identify the word's phonemes and match it to a lexeme. It checks to see if the lexeme has been processed and stored before and is therefore available. The similarity of a new word in L2 to a known word in L1 is important to how the brain assesses and acquires the new word. It seems that this type of assessment and discrimination process can only operate efficiently within the same lexical processing network. Differences in the speaker's level of proficiency can play a role in the speed with which the speaker can perform the rehearsal. A learner with a low level of proficiency might need more time to process a word when a transfer between L1 and L2 takes place. A highly proficient speaker would be able to process a new word faster, because that speaker already has more lexemes stored in long-term memory that might help identify the new word. Yet, the fMRI showed a separate set of neuroanatomical circuits for speakers who had acquired the L2 after the age of ten. The only conclusion is that the second circuit was used to grammatically encode the words.

Some support that speakers who acquire the L2 early in life use the same circuit when grammatically encoding words comes from an fMRI study by Willms et al. (2011). Their sixteen participants spoke Spanish as L1 and had acquired English before the age of seven or concurrently with Spanish, and were rated as having a high level of proficiency. They were presented with twenty-four English nouns, twenty-four Spanish nouns, twenty-four English verbs, and twenty-four Spanish verbs. After each presentation, they had to grammatically encode the word, if necessary. For example, they saw the words "one window" on a screen and on the next screen they saw "two ... " They were told to complete the sentence with the same word from the previous screen. In this case, the answer was "windows," indicating the plural. Likewise, they saw the words "él manda" [he commands] followed by "tú ... " The answer was "mandas," as Spanish pronoun-verb agreement requires an "s" for the second person singular "tú." Six of the twenty-four nouns and six of the twenty-four verbs were counterparts and presented in both languages; for example, the counterpart to "window" in Spanish was "ventana." The other words were semantically related in both languages. Participants had to speak the words out loud. Speaking poses problems for fMRI scans as the movement of the jaw distorts the imaging. Nevertheless, Willms et al. found that, when uttering the grammatically encoded words in either language, the same brain regions were active. Most notable was the high activation levels of the left posterior middle temporal gyrus – that is, part of the temporal lobe – when processing verbs. This is between Wernicke's area (left posterior superior temporal gyrus) and the hippocampus.

We cannot overlook the fact that the tasks of grammatically encoding the participants had to carry out were simple. Future studies need to analyze more complex tasks of sentence processing. For example, in German, constructing a relative clause requires not only using a relative pronoun that impacts the word order, but often using a preposition that is linked to a case, resulting in having to change the article (and sometimes the ending) of the noun. The problem then is to compare this type sentence to that of another language with equal grammatical complexity.

Grammar

Two arguments can be made in support of the theory that two circuits are used in the process of grammatical coding when the L2 is acquired later in life. The first argument is that the encoding of morphemes is quite complex.

The distinction of system morphemes proposed by Myers-Scotton and Jake (2000) is quite helpful when we describe the process with which one acquires another language. The distinction predicts that ESL learners produce early system morphemes such as plural "-s" with more accuracy than bridge system morphemes such as possessive "-s," and they produce bridge system morphemes with more accuracy than late system morphemes such as 3.P.Sg. Present Tense "-s." This is due to the fact that morphological markers for early system and bridge morphemes are activated at the lemma level of the lexeme, whereas the morphological markers for late morphemes are activated at a later stage of processing the lexeme. Therefore there is less chance for error in early system and bridge morphemes, as the learner has time to attach them properly, whereas the likelihood of error increases in late morphemes as the learner runs out of time before the late system morpheme can be accurately processed. These distinctions among different types of morphemes and how they are processed are naturally learned by the child who grows up with two languages. Consequently, the child uses one circuit. However, for the speaker who acquires another language at a later age (as in the case of the Kim et al., 1997 study that looked at learners between the ages of ten to twelve), the complexity inherent in the process of attachment in various types of morpheme is rather difficult to learn and does not allow the learner to use the same neuroanatomical circuit. Consequently, the learner develops a different neuroanatomical circuit for use in the new language.

The second argument is that grammatical rules are unique to a language and thus require a different system. For example, the form of a verb in German changes with its position in a sentence, which in some cases depends on other verbs: "Ich laufe nach Hause" [I run home] changes when the verb is moved to the end of the sentence, because of a modal verb, to "Ich will nach Hause laufen" [I want to run home]. The position and the form "laufen" is different compared to "run." Therefore it is only natural to expect that the brain must use two circuits in the process of grammatically encoding the words of two separate languages, unless the speaker acquired the two languages with equal practice from infancy. In such cases, the circuit in Broca's area allows for more variation because the brain itself is still in development. Such fluency and variation in the young developing brain also account for the example of code switches in the three-year-old who said "schraubing."

In order to compare early and late acquisition of a second language, Wartenburger et al. (2003) used fMRI to carry out a study with thirty-two healthy adults who spoke Italian as L1 and German as L2. They were divided into two groups, based on whether they had learned German early (before the age of six) or later (after the age of twelve, on average at the age of eighteen or nineteen). The participants were students living in Germany at the time. Both groups were proficient in L2, as determined by standard tests on German as a foreign language. For one of the experiments, they were asked to judge ninety sentences in German and ninety in Italian that had grammatical and semantic errors; for example, "Das Reh erschießt den Jäger" [the deer shoots the hunter]. They signaled an error by pressing a button. The early acquisition group did not show higher activation when carrying out semantic and grammatical tasks in German compared to Italian; however, the late acquisition group did, particularly in Broca's area. Interestingly, the late acquisition group performed as well as the early acquisition group on the test, although they used more energy (as shown in the extra activation) to achieve the result. The research also showed that when the participants judged lexical errors, the early acquisition and late acquisition groups (both highly proficient) activated the same region of the brain: the middle frontal gyrus that is part of the frontal lobe. This is not where Broca's area is located. However, this is where the executive control function directs attention to an incoming word and thereby indicates that the word should be processed in the phonological loop, which is part of Broca's area. When they were asked to judge grammatical errors, however, both groups activated all of the frontal lobe, including Broca's area, where phonemes, lexemes, and morphemes interact. The late acquisition group, however, did not perform as well as the early acquisition group, even though they showed higher levels of activation in Broca's area. One interpretation of this data is that they activated another circuit to judge the grammatical errors and, although they spent much energy doing so, it was not as successful as the early acquisition group, who only used one circuit. As usual there are problems with the study, despite the excellent design. Pressing a button on a recognition task is not the same as processing a word to be spoken. Also, testing errors in sentences activates many words, so it is impossible to distinguish between word groups. To test the errors in a sentence, for example, "Das Reh erschießt den Jäger" [the deer shoots the hunter], the participant combines lexical and grammatical errors, as the correct sentence could be "Der Jäger erschießt das Reh" [the hunter shoots the deer; lexically correct] or "Das Reh wird von dem Jäger erschossen" [the deer is shot by the hunter; grammatically correct]. Furthermore, the grammatical errors were a combination of morphology and syntax. Although that does reflect actual speech, it makes it difficult to analyze the results of the study to determine the precise way in which the brain encoded morphemes.

In a 2007 study using EEG, Chen, Shu, Liu, Zhao and Li analyzed learners' knowledge of grammar. Eighteen learners of English who spoke Chinese as their L1 had to judge whether or not sentences were correct. They had acquired English at the age of twelve and were considered a "late acquisition group." Forty-two sentences were presented word by word on a screen, and learners had to press a button once the complete sentence had been shown to indicate their decision. All sentences had subject-verb agreement violations; for example, "The price of the cars are too high." The same sentences were presented to native speakers of English, who also had to decide whether or not the sentences were correct. The study compared the electric waveforms of the "late acquisition group" to the ones of the native speakers. The waveforms were different. As mentioned in Chapter 2, "Memory, Language and the Brain," EEG studies have a time delay: the point of measurement at the scalp is not where the activity occurs inside the brain. Therefore, the electric waveform might be influenced by other factors, such as the central executive directing, dividing, or switching attention. We need to be cautious when interpreting results of EEG studies when it comes to language acquisition. However, this might be another indication that processing grammar requires two systems when the

L2 is acquired later in life, in particular when rules are substantially different between languages.

In summary, there is some indication to suggest that, in order to process words, a speaker largely uses one circuit regardless of the age of acquisition. However, in order to process grammar, the learner who has acquired the second language later in life must rely on two circuits. It is possible that by the time a learner is between six to eight years old when acquiring another language for the first time, s/he must begin to develop a second circuit in order to process certain aspects of grammar in that language. This has to do with certain complexities of grammar, as well as the fact that children at that age start to develop strategies to assist their learning. For example, in one cognitive strategy the learner may draw on prior knowledge to assist him or her to code words with the correct morphemes and to put them in the correct word order. However, in order to be successful, the speaker must have knowledge of the grammar rules, and must employ this knowledge properly. This is confirmed by reports that students who learn a language at college or university for the first time can achieve a great vocabulary (especially if the student goes abroad for six months or longer) but still make grammatical errors. For example, those who learn German as another language tend to make errors when they use late system morphemes to conjugate verbs because, in German, verbs are conjugated in relation to every pronoun (for example, 1.P.Sg. "Ich trinke Kaffee" [I drink coffee] is different than 3.P.Sg. "Er trinkt Kaffee" [He drinks coffee] or 3.P.Pl. "Sie trinken Kaffee" [They drink coffee].

Researchers of multiple language acquisition – that is, those who study polyglots or learners of several languages – argue that if learners start to acquire another language later (past twelve years of age) and use two circuits for grammatical processing – one for the first language and one for the new language – they keep using the circuit of the new language for all other languages they learn as well. Cenoz, Hufeisen, and Jessner (2003) have carried out groundbreaking work, although more research needs to be done in this area. In particular, researchers have not yet studied learners with different levels of proficiency. In other words, while beginners might use the network of L2 for acquiring L3, once they become more proficient in L3 they might use a direct L1-to-L3 connection in order to acquire more words. In addition, the similarity of the languages learned (L1 to L2, as well as L2 to L3 and L1 to L3) might play a role in what circuits are used.

When we think about theories of how words are processed, we have already considered the argument that it is inefficient for the brain to use more than one set of neuroanatomical circuits, in particular when we look at how the process of word acquisition and recall sets in motion: neurons fire simultaneously and converge (Pulvermüller, 1996; Singer, 2006; Tranel and Damasio, 2002); attention lights up working memory to zoom in on the incoming information

(Postle, 2006); the loop binds the word's sounds, supported by an underlying neural process (Buchsbaum and D'Esposito, 2008). To argue that there are two sets, we must ask how each set would know when to spring into action. It seems unlikely, given that lexemes and phonemes already carry language specific information.

The study by Kim and his colleagues was indeed remarkable, particularly for its time (in 1997!), for showing that differences among proficient bilingual speakers depended on the speaker's initial age of acquisition: participants who had acquired two languages early in life used one circuit for both languages, and those who had acquired the L2 later used two circuits. These circuits were found in Broca's area and can be attributed to grammatical encoding. In the section on neuroimaging, we learned that spatial resolution does not yet allow us to analyze whether there is variation within the language faculties when processing L2 and L1. However, with technological improvements we may soon be able to learn more about these circuit(s) in Broca's area, which will in turn allow us to learn more about the interplay of lexemes, phonemes, and morphemes.

7 Spacing

Spaced Repetition

When acquiring a new word in another language, the goal is to commit that word to long-term memory so it can be actively recalled and used later. A synapse that creates permanent access needs to be formed. This takes time, unless the word is fast-tracked due to heightened activation. Sometimes we cannot wait that long and need to learn new words immediately, for example, when going on vacation the following week or writing a vocabulary test. It is helpful to distinguish between long-term memory and short-term gains. We know that learning new words in intervals of repetition assists in the acquisition process. The question is how to space these intervals. The experiments with the sea slug *Aplysia* (Kandel, 2006) showed that its reflex to protect the gills was not modified if one stimulus took place but that five stimuli were necessary to change its behavior. If the stimulus was repeated with no pauses, *Aplysia*'s reaction lasted for up to a day; if the stimulus was repeated with pauses, it lasted up to four weeks. Although it is a bit of a stretch to go from *Aplysia* to acquiring words in another language, it is a starting point, leading to more detailed questions, such as:

- How long should the pauses in between each repetition be?
- How often does a word need to be repeated?
- Do we need to use different intervals for long-term memory compared to short-term gains?
- What is the overall time frame?

These questions have been debated for the past forty years to discover two things. First, the approach of repeating words within one learning session of seconds or minutes is substantially different than repeating words over multiple learning sessions in a period of days. Second, the point of testing plays a role. This is the point in time when participants in a study are asked to recall words after they have been repeated. Previous studies carried out in this area did not choose the same point of testing. Therefore, researchers often reported inconclusive or contradictory results.

If we take into account how words are processed in our brain, there are three factors any study investigating spacing intervals needs to take into account:

- speed
- rehearsal and repetition
- distraction.

The speed that a person can record a word into memory is linked to our capacity to direct, divide, and switch attention, a key process of working memory that demands much energy (Baddeley, 2007). As Skehan (1998, 2009a) explains in the limited capacity model, the brain's resources to process incoming and outgoing information are limited and therefore need to be allocated. The speed is also linked to the group that the word belongs to. The factors that determine the word group are length, similarity, and emotional connotation. Depending on these factors, a word might be fast-tracked into long-term memory or need a lot of time to be discriminated.

With regard to rehearsal, we need to make an important distinction between rehearsal and repetition. The phonological loop rehearses a word in a matter of a few hundred milliseconds: phonemes and lexemes need to be matched (Baddeley, 2007) to establish a form-to-meaning relationship (Nation, 2001). The form-to-meaning relationship is one of several aspects of what it means to know a word. It is also the starting point. If we only know parts of the word's form and meaning, it affects our ability to recall a word and thereby the fluency, accuracy, and complexity of speech. In order to remember a word, we often have to encounter the word more than once. The word needs to be repeated so it can be rehearsed again in the phonological loop. Researchers attempt to find out how often a word should be repeated and what type of interval should be used so that it will eventually be committed to long-term memory. Should it be repeated several times on the same day or spread out over a few days or longer? If it is spread out, should it be repeated every second day or should there be an expanded spacing pattern, such as repetition after one day, four days, and ten days?

In order to interrupt the rehearsal process and start a new set of repetitions, distraction items are used, in particular when words are learned in the same learning sessions. A good example is reciting all the US presidents in reverse order. This stops the processing of the words being studied, which is necessary in order to start a new rehearsal process when the word is repeated. However, when we refer to neurophysiology, we find that recently processed information can be reactivated relatively easily. Kandel (2006) demonstrated this when he explored how neurotransmitters transmit information from one neuron to the next in the sea slug *Aplysia*. Although distraction items are used in studies when testing the recall of words, we need to take into consideration how much time has passed since the word was last rehearsed. If words are tested minutes after the encounter, the loop is still active. At that point, it is difficult to say if a permanent record has been created. In fact, that might depend on the word group, as some words are fast-tracked and others are not. What is tested then is whether or not the loop is still active but not if words have been committed to long-term memory. Second language learners need to recall words days, weeks, and months after they have been acquired. Therefore, we need to make a distinction between recalling a word minutes or days later (short-term gains) or several weeks later (long-term memory), after the brain has initially processed the word. Summarizing research on spacing intervals, Roediger and Karpicke (2010) pointed out that many studies in the past did not make that distinction.

In general, the idea of spaced repetition is simple: the incoming information needs to be repeated and in between each repetition there needs to be a pause to give the memory a chance to process the information. Studies in this area have been carried out since the 1970s. Studies on sleep support the fact that information not only needs to be repeated but needs a break in between repetitions. More than sixty years ago, Sokoloff and his colleagues (1953) wanted to find out how much oxygen the brain uses when it is thinking or solving difficult tasks. Solokoff had one of his students carry out those difficult tasks and he measured the oxygen level in the student's brain. He also measured the same student's oxygen level at rest. Surprisingly, he discovered that the brain does not use more oxygen when it is thinking compared to when it is resting. It was a discovery that had everyone puzzled but was then forgotten for decades. However, in 2001, an article published by Raichle and his colleagues described the same phenomena as Sokoloff and his colleagues (Raichle et al., 2001). Of course, by then the technology had changed. Raichle and his colleagues monitored the brains of forty-nine participants using PET as well as fMRI. The results from the PET study were quite interesting. PET measures blood flow by injecting a radioactive substance into the bloodstream and monitoring which region of the brain it travels to. The substance travels to the region that is most active at the time because it reacts to the chemical influx of the activation. Each of the participants in this study, all adults and native speakers of English, had to carry out a variety of cognitive tasks, including language tasks. Single English nouns were played over speakers one by one so that participants could hear them. Then the participants had to think of a verb that was appropriate in meaning with respect to the given noun and say it out loud. This method had been used before (Petersen et al., 1989). Another language task utilized the same method except that nouns were presented visually and not aurally. In this case, however, the verbs that participants thought of still had to be said out loud. Raichle and his team measured the brain activity of the participants carrying out these tasks as well as the brain activity of the same participants when they were resting with their eyes closed. The PET showed that some areas of the brain remained very active when eyes were closed, but other areas of the brain were not as active. The most notable inactive brain areas were parts of the prefrontal cortex and the upper part of the limbic system. The researchers proposed that, in the resting state, the brain switches to a default mode.

What does the brain do when it is in default mode? More research needs to be carried out in this area, but currently some researchers seem to think that the brain reviews the information it had received before it went into the resting state. We know that the dorsolateral prefrontal region rests during REM sleep (Muzur, Pace-Schott, and Hobson, 2002) while the main part of the limbic system is quite active. We can deduce that, while the executive control of working memory (which coordinates attention to incoming information) rests, and consequently no new information is attended to, information that entered the brain before sleep – including emotions – is processed again. Since the hippocampus sits deep down in the limbic system, it is possible that to some degree the record of a word is reviewed. In addition to reviewing, the brain might also sort out information that is considered important from information it received that is considered unimportant, strengthen the important information, and link it to other previously existing information. How, exactly, that happens still needs to be investigated but likely it has to do with the synchronization of neurons. In default mode, circuits are activated to coordinate the information (Raichle, 2010, 2011). This is supported by the fact that, out of all the neurons we have, more are involved in reviewing information within the brain than in processing new incoming information.

Applying the findings of these studies on sleep to learning new words, we can argue that it is indeed helpful, not only to repeat words but to do so with a spacing effect. The spacing effect provides a break in between repetitions that allows the brain to go into default mode. Simply said, it might be a good idea to sleep on it. For example, if you encounter a new word today and then again tomorrow, there is a higher chance that the word will eventually be stored in long-term memory than if you were to encounter that word two or three times within an hour. In a study with 191 students at the University of Lübeck, Born and his colleagues tested this hypothesis (Wilhelm et al., 2011). Students, who were native speakers of German, had to learn forty English word associates. They were divided into six groups: one group studied the word associates for one hour in the evening and was allowed to sleep afterward; one group studied the word associates for one hour in the evening and was not allowed to sleep afterward; one group studied the word associates for one hour in the morning and was not allowed to sleep afterward. Half of the students in each group were told that they would be tested nine hours after the learning phase; the other half of the students were not given that information. A post-questionnaire was used to exclude the results of students who indicated that they had suspected that a test was coming, despite not being told that they would be tested. After the learning phase, each group played a short computer game as a distractor for fifteen minutes. The groups who were not allowed to sleep continued to play board and other games with the experimenter. The retention test showed that, for those students who were not told that they were tested, it did not matter if they were allowed to sleep, or not, after the learning phase. Their scores on the word association task did not differ much. However, for those who were told that a test was coming, it did matter. The group who was allowed to sleep outperformed the two groups that were not allowed to sleep.

All in all, more studies have been carried out in cognitive psychology than in second language acquisition. Studies in cognitive psychology are often set in a lab environment in order to control as many factors as possible. Participants are shown words, pictures, or names using different types of spaced repetitions. The idea is to isolate words so they can be processed efficiently. Studies in second language acquisition often use a different environment. These studies are mostly carried out in a classroom setting, to reflect the situation where one would talk to other people. Words are acquired in various texts and contexts. Both types of approaches have advantages and disadvantages. Studies carried out in a lab do not resemble actual communication, whereas in classroom studies a researcher does not have full control over the participants' interactions, bringing with this the chance that some unknown factor will influence the results. An alternative is to use a crossover study which uses the methods developed in one discipline (cognitive psychology) and applies them to another (second language acquisition).

In the following section, we will look at studies that have been carried out in both of these disciplines, discuss their pros and cons, and see if we can find some middle ground that leads us to answer our questions. Usually, these studies use participants that are students enrolled in a college or university.

Testing of Spacing Effects

One of the first studies attempting to measure recall was by Turvey, Brick, and Osborne (1970). The study was carried out in cognitive psychology. This was not that surprising, since the study of memory was an emerging line of inquiry at the time. In the first experiment, three groups of undergraduate students had to listen to five different consonant sounds. One group had to recall the consonant sounds after five seconds; one group, after ten seconds; and one group, after twenty-five seconds. Participants recalling after twenty-five seconds recalled as many sounds correctly as subjects recalling after five or ten seconds. At the time, this was quite a surprise, because it was assumed that the phonological loop could only hold information for up to two seconds. We now know that it can hold information for up to two minutes. In a supplementary experiment, each group carried out a recall test fifteen seconds after the first test. In that test, the group with the twenty-five-second delay recalled more sounds than the other two groups. We now know that a short delay of five seconds might result in automatic processing. Therefore, the sounds that needed to be processed by the participants of the five-second-delay group did not receive enough attention, resulting in a lack of "elaborate rehearsal" (Craik and Lockhart, 1972) and poorer recall.

However, it has been a long road to get to where we are today. Many studies have been carried out, each of them improving the methodology and learning from previous studies. I will only focus on a few of them that help us understand the spacing effect. In the field of cognitive psychology, Landauer and Bjork carried out a study on spaced repetition in 1978. Their method was quite simple: they had students play cards. At the State University of New York at Stony Brook, students had to remember sixteen cards that were part of a deck of fifty-two. Each card had a picture of a face with a name underneath. Students looked at each card in the deck for nine seconds. Twelve cards each appeared four times within the deck and the other four cards were interleaved as distraction items. After going through the deck of cards once, students went through the deck three more times. The distraction cards were spaced using five different intervals. The three most important intervals were:

- a massed pattern with no distraction cards in between (i.e., 0-0-0): a name/face card was repeated four times followed by the next name/face card, which was repeated four times and the next name/face card also repeated four times.
- a uniform pattern (i.e., 4-4-4): name/face card – four distraction cards – same name/face card – four distraction cards – same name/face card – four distraction cards.
- an expanded pattern (i.e., 1-4-10): name/face card – one distraction card – same name/face card – four distraction cards – same name/face card – ten distraction cards.

This idea to repeat the same item within the same learning session stems from the so-called "Hebb Effect," named after the Canadian psychologist Donald O. Hebb. Hebb (1949, 1961) presented his subjects with lists of nine digits. On some of the lists, every third digit was repeated to create a pattern. It turned out that subjects remembered the lists that had a pattern better than the lists that did not have a pattern. On Hebb's lists, the pattern was regular (every third item), with at least one item in between to create a break. He did not use other patterns – for example, three items in a row, or an expanded pattern such as repeating the third, sixth, and tenth item. That was Landauer and Bjork's (1978) innovative approach.

The question was: Which kind of interval works best? Each card deck that students went through was pre-sorted so that it contained each of the different spacing patterns. After students went through the card decks for the last time, they had to listen to a thirty-minute lecture followed by a test of recall on the twelve cards. In the test, they saw the face cards and had to recall the names. The distraction of the lecture was necessary to counter the effect of automaticity by making sure that the processing of the name/face cards had stopped. This ensured that the recall tests actually assessed what had been remembered and not what was still being processed. In essence, this method is still used today, although it is a bit more advanced now with the use of computers. The results of Landauer and Bjork's (1978) study showed that the expanded pattern brought about the highest recall rates, the uniform pattern had the second highest, and the massed pattern had the lowest recall rates. Neither Turvey, Brick, and Osborne (1970) nor Landauer and Bjork tested recall after a longer time period had passed. Their tests were done shortly after the learning phase. Testing students the following day would have been interesting due to the studies on sleep, which showed how a default mode sets in when the brain "rests." During this state the brain reviews some information and discards other information (Raichle et al., 2001).

The method Landauer and Bjork (1978) used does not exactly reflect what happens when encountering a new word in another language. Their study was not designed to test that; it was designed to study memory. When encountering and hopefully acquiring a new word in another language, there are two differences. First, we often encounter new words because we hear them and not because we see them, as with the playing cards. Studies in cognitive psychology often present words visually but not aurally or both. Second, we are often in a situation where we need to recall words we learned days, weeks, months, or even years, later. Successfully recalling words or names/faces thirty minutes after the encounter does not necessarily mean they can be recalled in the following days. Nevertheless, the result that an expanded interval leads to higher recall rates was accepted for a while not only when describing memory but also when learning vocabulary. In the field of second language acquisition, flashcard systems based on expanded intervals had been developed since the 1960s and were used in language classrooms to learn as many new words as possible (Leitner, 1972; Pimsleur, 1967). The development of these flashcards was welcomed by language instructors, who had observed that students not only needed to repeat information, but needed to do so over longer periods of time. The expanded interval technique used in these flashcard systems was spread over a period of days, thereby changing the approach from practicing a word within one learning session to practicing it over multiple sessions. We discuss these flashcard systems in more detail below.

More than twenty-five years later, Carpenter and DeLosh (2005) carried out a study based on spaced repetition that was similar to what Landauer and Bjork had conducted in 1978. However, in this case, Carpenter and DeLosh presented name/face cards on a computer, increased the number of items to be tested to thirty, as well as eighteen distraction items, and after each item was presented for six seconds (instead of nine seconds), the three repetitions took place. The distraction items were spaced 0-0-0 (massed), 3-3-3 (uniform), and 1-3-5 (expanded). When students finished, they were asked to name as many US states as possible in five minutes, which served as the distraction task. Immediately afterward, students had to recall the names of the faces on the cards. Results confirmed that the lowest recall rate was at the massed interval. However, no differences between the uniform and expanded spacing were found. In a second experiment, the expanded pattern was stretched to a 3-5-7 interval, but the recall rate was still similar to that of the uniform interval. Although Landauer and Bjork, as well as Carpenter and DeLosh, carried out tests shortly after the learning phase, Landauer and Bjork's result (that the expanded interval leads to higher recall rates) was not verified by Carpenter and DeLosh's study.

Between 1978 and 2005, there were other studies confirming that the massed interval does not work very well. This is supported by how memory is formed, with the modification/formation of new synapses as well as by the workings of the phonological loop. If a word is simply being repeated with no pauses in between, the processing becomes automatic. The automatic processing leads to less activity and therefore phonemes and lexemes are not discriminated sufficiently. That makes it difficult to create a record of the word. This reminds us of the *Aplysia* case. When *Aplysia* was stimulated repeatedly with no pauses in between stimuli, its reflex reaction lasted for no longer than a day, but when the stimulation was done repeatedly with pauses, the reaction lasted for up to four weeks. In that case, a chemical process was triggered, which led to forming a new synapse that stored the recorded information permanently. Therefore, the information could be recalled later.

This brings us back to two points that are important when acquiring new words in another language. First is the point of testing (Roediger and Karpicke, 2010). If a test is administered minutes after the learning phase, there is a chance that the loop is still in action and, even if it is not, the recent practice sessions make it easy to restart the loop. Consequently, any differences in processing are difficult to determine. Second, the brain needs to rest to digest the information it has encountered (Raichle et al., 2001). This implies that testing should be carried out at different points in time, such as a few minutes after the learning phase, the next day, a few days after the learning phase, and/or a few weeks after the learning phase. In a review article summarizing research on spaced repetition, Balota, Duchek, and Logan (2007) take the practical view that it is important to have the same participants recall words at least twice: once shortly after the last practice session, and once much later. In their review, they draw our attention to two studies that revealed exactly that problem. The first study was conducted with three groups: young healthy adults, older healthy adults, and older patients impaired by early stages of Alzheimer's (Balota et al., 2006). Each group learned English-English word associates such as "ground-cold." Each pair was presented once and then cued for recall by showing only the first word (for example, "ground") and asking for the associate (for example, "cold"). In the first experiment, participants received no feedback. If the response was incorrect, participants moved to the next word. In the second experiment, feedback was given. If the response was correct, they moved to the next word. If not, the correct response was provided. Three different intervals were used: a massed, a uniform, and an expanded interval. After the learning phase, a five-minute distraction task was administered followed by a test. In both experiments, the test showed that using the massed interval led to the lowest recall rates. No differences were recorded between the use of the uniform and expanded interval. The second study compared only two groups: young, healthy adults and older, healthy adults (Logan and Balota, 2008). The design of the study was similar to the Balota et al. study (2006). However, in addition to carrying out an immediate test, another test was administered twenty-four hours later. The immediate test confirmed that using the uniform and expanded interval resulted in similar recall rates, whereas using the massed interval resulted in lower recall rates. The test after a twenty-four-hour delay showed that all of the scores for all three intervals dropped. They dropped the most for the massed interval, the second most for the expanded interval, and the least for the uniform interval.

Wagner, Maril, and Schacter (2000) carried out a study on spacing intervals using fMRI technology. The students, who were divided into two groups, were shown a list of words and were told they would be tested later. The first group saw the same list again minutes later (massed repetition) and the second group saw the list again a day later (space repetition). The fMRI showed that, in the first group, the prefrontal cortex of the left hemisphere (rehearsal) was less active. If words are repeated too close together, the second rehearsal is automatic and the activity of the rehearsal is reduced. Consequently, phonemes are not necessarily matched to a lexeme. Although that provides evidence that using massed spacing is the least effective method, it does not solve the question as to whether uniform or expanded spacing is more beneficial.

Spaced repetition has been tested with patients who suffer from memory loss. A general problem with applying this technique with patients is that they have to learn the technique itself. Although it is simple for healthy subjects to repeat words following a certain schedule, patients suffering from memory loss find it much more difficult. The reason why this technique has been attempted with patients is that it provides error-free feedback. Patients associate techniques with the information they need to learn (Wilson et al., 1994). If the experimenters were to make use of errors in the feedback – for example, by explaining the type of error – patients might start to remember the error but not the correct word. Instead, the spaced repetition simply reinforces the correct information and in turn that information might help patients. Out of the many studies carried out with patients suffering from Alzheimer's, most of them had the patients learn activities such as how to use a calendar or locate objects. However, in a study on words (Abrahams and Camp, 1993), two Alzheimer's patients were trained to recall names of common objects. Nine objects were used in the study. In a pre-test, the two patients could not name these objects. Two of the objects were the objects to be relearned and the other seven objects were used as controls. Patients participated in three training sessions over a one-week period. They were shown an object and asked to name it. If they were able to do so, the object was shown again five seconds later and they were asked again. If they were not able to do so, they were told the name of the object and had to repeat it. Then they were shown the object again five seconds later. For the control items, that was all that was done, but for the two objects to be relearned, this technique continued by either increasing (if the patient could name the object) or decreasing (if the patient could not name the object) the time interval between asking the patients to name the objects. Initially, increases followed a spaced interval of ten, twenty, and thirty seconds. If the patient was able to name the object after the thirty-second interval, the intervals were increased further to see how much time could pass until the patient was no longer able to name the object. While patient 1 was able to name one of the items after a time interval of five minutes, patient 2 was able to do so with both items. One week after the last training session, both patients were tested again. They were shown all nine items. They could not name the seven control items, but were able to name both of the items they had learned.

Short-term Gains vs. Long-term Memory

We still need to answer the question of whether we should use a particular interval (uniform or expanded) for short-term gains or for committing words to long-term memory. In regards to the neurophysiology, either way a synapse is created. We learned in Chapter 3, "Synaptic Connections," that information can be processed temporarily or accessed permanently. In the later case, a synaptic connection is created. The difference is that the synaptic connection for short-term gains is very fragile because it is built quickly; it can collapse if no further construction is carried out. Recalling the word a few more times constructs a record of the word that is then committed to long-term memory. This construction is solid and will last longer. How does this translate into actual times? Short-term gains are when information can be recalled for up to a few days after that information was processed last. It should not be confused with word echoing, during which words are repeated back immediately after they are heard. In word echoing no synapse is formed. Long-term memory is associated with the ability to recall words several weeks, or even months, after they were first encountered. We need to keep in mind that the words committed to long-term memory need maintenance as well. If the record is not updated once in a while, the synaptic bridge can fall apart like any other.

Is the distinction between short-term gains and long-term memory with regard to spacing intervals helpful for second language learners? In theory, it is. If one of the intervals is more efficient for short-term gains, it might be used when studying for a vocabulary test. If a language learner wants to build his or her vocabulary over the duration of a semester, a different interval might lead to higher recall rates. A priority for language teachers should be to educate language learners about what type of spacing to use in each learning situation. We will return to this in Chapter 9, "Learning and Teaching."

Two researchers who have performed many studies on second language vocabulary acquisition are Laufer and Hulstijn. Most of their subjects were students learning English in either Israel or the Netherlands. Some of the studies focused on production, which is important in the context of repeating words. Hulstijn and Laufer (2001) argued that every speaker with the need to use a word in a sentence has to search to find the word that expresses a certain concept, evaluate that word compared to other words, and recognize differences. In each of these three phases, the word in question receives attention. Once the word has been found and checked, it is activated. Hulstijn and Laufer's studies show the importance of producing words when learning them. Students should write or say the word they are trying to learn as opposed to just reading the word or repeating it subvocally in their heads.

A few years later, Webb (2005) carried out a study confirming that, when learning words, tasks requiring production result in higher retention rates than tasks that focus solely on comprehension. Participants in this study were Japanese undergraduate students of English. Twenty non-words and a Japanese translation were presented to them. The non-words had been created to resemble actual English words and were pre-tested so that students actually thought they were real words. Non-words were used to avoid the possibility of any participant recognizing one of the English words used in the study. Participants had to carry out two learning tasks. For ten non-words, they had to read three sentences per word (reading comprehension) and, for each of the other ten non-words, they had to write a sentence in English using that word (writing production). Webb did not tell them that they would be tested on those same words afterward. Several tests were carried out as soon as both tasks had been completed. Each test had a comprehension and a production component. For example, participants listened to the non-words and either had to identify them from a list of four given words or had to write them down. In another test, students had to either pick the correct use of that word from three sentences (only one of the sentences being correct) or they had to use the non-words in a sentence. Webb arranged the order of the tests so that no words were tested in direct succession. Results of these tests showed that participants scored higher on the comprehension tests, such as identifying or picking non-words, than on the production tests, such as writing a word down or using the word in a sentence. These results came as no surprise because, in a test on comprehension, the word is given in a context of other words that are all previously acquired and known to the learner. These can act as clues to assist in processing the lexeme and phonemes of the word that is being tested because they provide meaning as well as narrow down the selection of the lexemes and phonemes that need to be discriminated. With fewer possibilities, there is less chance of error. However, in a production test, the speaker has to create the context. Many lexemes and phonemes are rehearsed to be matched, bearing a greater chance of error. That type of test also requires more energy. Webb's study showed that, in all tests (receptive and productive), participants scored higher on the ten words they had previously learned by writing compared to those they had learned by reading.

In a recent study, Barcroft (2015) confirmed Webb's (2005) results. Barcroft gave undergraduate students in Mexico City learning English as a foreign language ten minutes to read a text that contained five words, which they were tested on immediately after they finished reading. They did not know they were being tested. They were simply told to read for meaning. For one group of thirty-seven students the five words, which occurred three times in the text passage, were presented with translations. For another group of thirty-seven students, the translation was provided the first time each of those words occurred in the text, and a blank space shown next to the word when it appeared in the text the second and third time. Students of that group were asked to fill in the blank by producing the word. Results of the vocabulary quiz carried out immediately after the study showed that this group performed much better than the group who did not have to produce those words.

When carrying out a writing task to learn a new word, it is necessary to differentiate between just writing the word down and writing the word down as part of a sentence. Producing an entire sentence with a new word can be very demanding. Not only does the newly acquired word need to be recalled, but also all of the other words in the sentence. Barcroft (2004) tested this in a study with learners of Spanish. In that study, learners saw twenty-four word-picture pairs. For half of the words, learners needed to create a sentence in Spanish containing the new word and write the sentence down. For the other half, learners needed to simply write down the new word. Three tests were carried out afterward where learners were shown the picture and had to write down the word. One test was carried out immediately after the learning phase, one was two days later, and the last test was one week later. On all three tests, students recalled more words that had been just written down without having to create a sentence. These results were later replicated by Wong and Pyun (2012), with learners of French and Korean.

What do we gather from these studies? When learning new words, we should take some time to process a new word and avoid putting too much demand on that process. Strain to this process can occur by attempting to recall many other words at the same time, even if those other words have been acquired already. In short, something that should be avoided when acquiring new words is to create long lists with many examples of how to use that word. This can be done once the word has been acquired but, even then, the number of examples should be kept to a minimum, since every word of every example needs to be processed along with it. This places a high demand on the phonological loop. Since resources are limited, the higher the demand is on the loop, the less processing capacity is available to deal with all of those examples. It is more likely to remember how to use a new word in one or two examples than in five or six.

In summary, the type of task used when acquiring new words is important. Specifically, one should not only rely on comprehension but employ a productive task. The productive task needs to be carefully chosen to avoid overburdening the language faculties. It needs to be a simple task, such as writing down the word. At a later phase, one or two example sentences can be processed comprehensively or productively. Furthermore, the spacing between repetitions is important, to ensure that the loop is not still actively rehearsing the word when it is encountered again. To confirm this, time needs to pass or a distraction needs to be created. Ideally, both of these factors are implemented. Any vocabulary program should take these factors into account.

Computerized Spacing

Most devices used for second language vocabulary learning, such as flashcards or computerized programs, ignore how words are processed in the brain. Most vocabulary programs do not distinguish between short-term gains and long-term memory nor do they contain productive tasks. However, they do provide lists of similar-sounding words or words of the same semantic group and use many examples to illustrate the words. Consequently, the discrimination process of phonemes and lexemes is more difficult for the loop, as well as Wernicke's area, to handle.

Flashcards have been around since the 1960s and 1970s. Pimsleur's (1967), as well as Leitner's "Die Lernkatei" (1972), used the concept of structured cyclical repetition. The concept was based on the principle of forgetting, which was influenced by the research of Ebbinghaus (1913). In the first trial of his self-experiments, Ebbinghaus memorized a collection of nonsense words. He then measured the seconds he saved when relearning the words in each subsequent trial, which took place after twenty minutes, one hour, nine hours, one day, two days, six days, and thirty-one days. He concluded that forgetting occurs within a few minutes after the first trial. In Leitner's "Lernkatei," the term to be learned is written on one side of a flashcard and the prompt on the other. Ideally, the daily input is determined by the size of a daily vocabulary learning routine. Leitner postulated that the daily input is limited to twelve to fifteen new words. However, we have to think about repeating words in the subsequent days after initial encounter. In fact, if we learn eight words per day we will acquire 5,000 words in less than two years. That might be more manageable, as on subsequent days the words that need to be repeated mix with new words. A learner puts the flashcards with each of those words in the first compartment of a six-compartment box and then takes them out one by one and attempts to memorize them. "Die Lernkartei" had five to six compartments of progressively larger sizes. It operated on the principle that repetition needed to take place through multiple learning sessions over a longer period of time such as days or even weeks. Once a word is remembered, the learner moves the flashcard of that word up to the next compartment. Incorrect ones drop back to, or remain in, the first compartment. The flashcard boxes have been used in the German school system for many years for learners of English as a Second Language. One issue with this system is that there has been no published research on how these flashcards are processed and handled. The learner determines if s/he has acquired a word successfully as well as when and how long s/he will practice.

During the nineties, Mondria and Mondria-de Vries (1994) developed a computer-assisted learning program incorporating the learning system of Leitner. The program was based on words from a textbook. Mondria and Mondria-de Vries advocated its use as a less time-consuming activity compared to the flashcard writing. In addition, the program featured sound files and images, which was something flashcards did not originally have. Yet again, no research was carried out. Students had to decide for themselves if they had learned the word or not. Around the same time, Oxford (1990) promoted a staggered learning technique in her renowned textbook. Based on teaching experience, she suggested that an item that needs to be memorized should be repeated using seven intervals: fifteen minutes, one hour, two hours, one day, four days, one week, and two weeks.

Ideally, we learn a word with its sound as well as an associative image and smell, the same way we would encounter that word in the country where the language we are learning is predominantly spoken. In our brain, hearing a word causes the phonemes of that word to go directly into the phonological loop. When reading a word, its phonemes have to be transcribed into a phonological code. That is an extra step that requires time. On the plus side, the visual code can assist in rehearsing the lexeme of that word. In order to create a record of a word, phonemes have to be matched to a lexeme, and information is recorded from the senses. From the olfactory bulb, occipital lobe, and auditory cortex, the enthornial and perirhinal cortices feed sensory information to the hippocampus. Therefore, processing a word with sounds, images, and smell supports building a synapse, committing that word to long-term memory.

In addition to presenting words with sounds and images, it is helpful to encounter a word with its translation, a definition, and/or sample sentences to acquire all aspects of form and meaning (Nation, 2001). However, one has to be careful as to how many examples are used. The advantage of a computer program is that information can be revealed upon request by the user. This gives the learner the option to decide how much of that information s/he wants to see at the same time or in succession (Nation, 2001). This is consistent with the theory of dynamic systems (Miller, 2002; Thelen, 2005; Thomas, 2001). Applied to language learning, the two systems of vocabulary and grammar compete with one another when building one's vocabulary. This has been shown with studies on lexical growth in children (Robinson and Mervis, 1998) but is equally relevant for adult second language learners at the beginner's level. The competition is avoided, because the information can be acquired in sequence. From a teaching perspective, providing several modalities (image, sound, sample sentences or definition, translation) has the advantage in that it caters to the preferred learning style of each student (Kim and Gilman, 2008; Oxford, 2003; Rimrott, 2010). Furthermore, a computer program can decide if a word has been successfully acquired. It can also provide feedback by presenting some or all of the information again.

In a series of experiments that I conducted with my graduate student (Schütze and Weimer-Stuckmann, 2010, 2011), we programmed a computerized vocabulary trainer with two algorithms – the first was for the uniform interval and the other was for the expanded interval – in order to investigate the relationship between those intervals and short-term gains vs. long-term memory. The trainer used all modalities described above to cater to every preferred learning style. Our vocabulary trainer also tracked which words had been acquired and which ones had to be repeated.

We carried out our research in an environment where the language being learned was not the one that was predominantly spoken in the country. That reflects a situation most people are in when learning another language. Our participants consisted of undergraduate students who were learning German for the first time at a West Coast university in Canada. This type of language learning environment minimized the chance that words were acquired by coincidence. Naturally, it was still possible for students to get in contact with German-speaking people or material that is in German by chatting or surfing on the internet, but it was quite uncommon for students to do so, due to being busy with other classes. To make sure, we used two questionnaires filled out by our participants. The first questionnaire was carried out before we ran the experiments and asked about the participants' language backgrounds. This was designed to avoid anyone participating that already knew some German. The second questionnaire was carried out after the experiments had been completed and asked participants if they had used any other techniques to study words. If so, they were asked which ones and what kind of contact they had to German-speaking sources throughout the experiments. Those who did use other techniques and/or had contact with Germans were excluded from the analysis.

The words that were used in the study were taken from the textbook of a beginner's German course. Every two weeks, students had to learn forty words. They did this five times (they go through five chapters of the textbook per term) for a total of ten weeks and 200 words. The procedure was very straightforward: students were given a schedule as when to practice the words.

The vocabulary trainer we developed presented words one at a time. The program integrated factors we considered essential when acquiring new words: each word was presented visually and aurally along with a translation, one sample sentence, and a productive task where students had to type in the new word every time they were asked to. Feedback was immediate. If the word was typed into the program correctly, the learner was directed to the next word. If it was incorrect, the learner was directed to review the information (image, audio, sample sentence, meaning) associated with that word, thereby receiving positive reinforcement.

At the end of every two weeks, students wrote a test for each chapter in which they were given an English word and had to write down the German word. We tested students at the beginning of the following week, so there were four days in between the last practice and the test. All in all, there were five chapter tests. In each of those, we tested twenty of the forty words, to avoid students guessing some answers.

Students were divided into two different groups. One group used a uniform schedule and the other group used an expanded schedule (Schütze and Weimer-Stuckmann, 2011). All participants encountered each word five times. The schedules were programmed into the vocabulary trainer. Students assigned to the uniform group had access to the trainer after the initial encounter where they could practice on day two, four, six, and eight. Students using the expanded interval had access to the trainer on day one (twice), day three, and day six. No distraction items were used, since the experiments of this study spanned over multiple sessions. Therefore, enough time had passed in between repetitions for the rehearsal process to start afresh by the time the words were encountered again. An exception was with the expanded interval group, who had two sessions on the first day, because that was the only time students were not allowed to sleep on it. However, those two sessions took place once in the morning and once in the evening so that students had plenty of distractions in between from attending other classes. The program allowed us to track which words students had practiced and at what time, to verify that they had followed the prescribed schedule of either the uniform or the expanded interval when studying all of the words.

The study consisted of several experiments: one set of experiments between September and December 2008 in "Beginning German I," and one set of experiments between January and April 2009 in "Beginning German II." All in all, we analyzed the results of 155 students (86 students in the fall of 2008 and 69 students in the spring of 2009). Initially, there were a total of 207 students. This occurred for two reasons: first, the two questionnaires (one on the language background of students and one on the techniques used; see above) showed that some students were not ideal candidates for the study; and, second, some students did not practice the words with the online program at the times they were supposed to. We were able to check this with the tracking function of the program. Students who take "Beginning German I" usually continue with "Beginning German II." The interval that each student started with (uniform vs. expanded) was kept for both courses, so a student who was in the uniform group in "Beginning German I" remained in the uniform group for "Beginning German II." This was done to be consistent and to be able to continue with further testing down the road.

After all the planning, programming, careful design, and data collection of many students, results showed that both interval groups were very successful in recalling words when tested four days after the last repetition. However, there was no statistically significant difference between the two interval groups. We repeated the study the following year, in the fall of 2009 and the spring of 2010 with a similar number of students. This time, students could practice the words up to four times. Results were still not statistically different when comparing the uniform group with the expanded group.

Of course, what we really wanted to know was what students remembered many weeks and months after the last practice. We carried out tests at the end of each term – that is, in December 2008, April 2009, December 2009, and April 2010. Each time, we tested fifty words, taking ten words from each chapter. We called it the first long-term retention test. The test was done two weeks after the last chapter vocabulary quiz. That meant that some of the words had last been rehearsed twelve weeks before (words from the first chapter) and some only two weeks before (words from the fifth chapter). Overall, students did not remember as many words as they did on the chapter tests, which was to be expected. Over time, some words had been forgotten. In all of these tests, students who had practiced with the uniform interval recalled more words than those who had practiced with the expanded interval. However, differences were not statistically significant.

Of course, we were not done yet. We did another test. We called it the second long-term retention test. It was carried out when participants came back to the university the following fall. For the students who had participated the previous fall, that meant a delay of nine months between the first long-term retention test and the second long-term retention test. For the students who had participated in the spring of that academic year, it meant a delay of five months. In this test, fifty words were tested. This time, we only chose five words from each chapter, because we now had words from ten chapters (five from each course) to deal with. We also did not want to make the test too long. This would have made it difficult for students to focus on the test for the entire duration. The results were statistically different. The retention rate of students who had practiced with the uniform interval was 83 percent and the retention rate of students who had practiced with the expanded interval was 59 percent. The statistics were done using analysis of variance (ANOVA) with a 95 percent confidence interval, eliminating very high and very low scores as well as taking into account variances from chapter to chapter. This meant that the results were reliable. However, a limitation of the second long-term retention test was that we did not know what students had done over the summer. In order to find out, they were asked to fill out another questionnaire asking about their contact with native speakers of German or travels in a German-speaking country, etc. Those who had contact were eliminated from the study. There were only a few students that we had to eliminate. That was a bit of a surprise, because we thought students would take the opportunity to go abroad to the country whose predominant language they had begun to learn. The reality was that most of our students had to work at various jobs during the summer in the hospitality industry (restaurants, cafés, hotels) or at summer camps or planting trees. When they came back to school in September, it was as if they were starting to learn German all over again.

In summary, our experiments showed that when words were encountered five times over a time frame of ten days, recall rates were high for short-term gains (days after last repetition) and less high for long-term memory (weeks after last repetition) when using either a uniform or expanded interval. However, in the very long term (months after the last repetition), having used the uniform interval seemed to be more beneficial. Figure 8 provides an overview of these spacing patterns.

We need to be aware, though, that practicing words five times is not the magic number of second language vocabulary acquisition. It worked in the context of this study with regard to the level of proficiency (beginner), the development phase of the learners (university undergraduate students), and learning

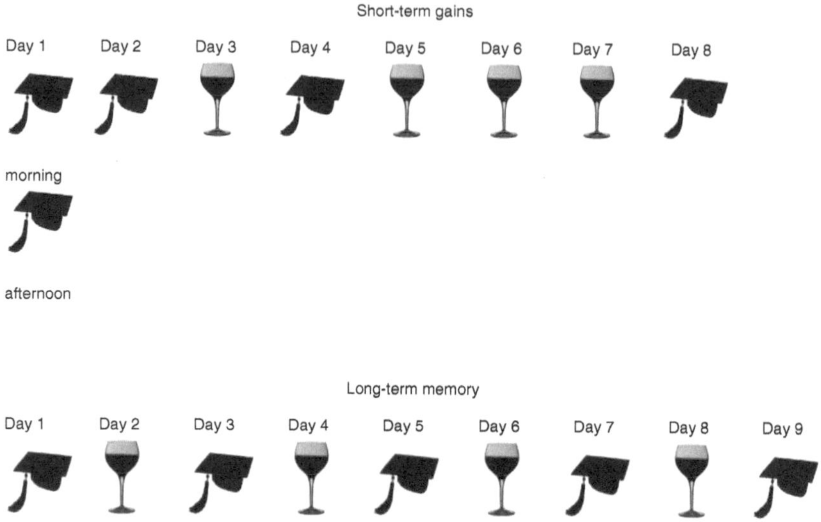

Figure 8. Optimized Spacing Patterns.

environment (language to be learned not predominantly spoken). If any of those factors change, a different number of repetitions and a different time frame might be needed. Furthermore, the languages tested (English/German) are closely related, belonging to the West Germanic language group. We need to consider that if learning a language that is substantially different from our L1 in orthography and phonetics – for example, if our L1 is English and we learn Japanese – the rehearsal process will need to be repeated more often.

In the post-study discussions, more questions were raised. What if we had tested the same day after the last repetition, as studies in cognitive psychology do? In that case, we would have included a distraction between the last repetition and the test. Would there have been differences between the expanded and uniform interval? Can we set up a study that will distinguish between different word categories or groups? For example, is there a difference between content and function words in relation to the uniform or expanded interval? Are longer and similar words indeed more difficult to process, and do they therefore need more than five practices? Are emotional words really fast-tracked? While my graduate student started a Ph.D. to look into how instructors think they teach second language vocabulary, I started a project attempting to answer these questions related to how words are processed in the brain. The results of this project are presented in Chapter 8, "Word Analysis."

The question of how instructors think they teach second language vocabulary is an interesting one. In a recent publication, Kornell and Bjork (2010) pointed out that there is a difference between how we learn and how we think we learn. The same can be said about teaching. In a series of experiments, Kornell and Bjork tested undergraduate students on how they judged their own learning. In one of the experiments, they gave the students two lists, each with twenty English-Swahili word pairs. Students had ten minutes to study the words. Each word was on a card presented on a computer screen. In the first trial, the Swahili word appeared for three seconds, disappeared, and then the English word appeared for three seconds. In the second and all subsequent trials, the Swahili word appeared for three seconds, disappeared, and then the students were asked to type in the English word. After that, the correct English word appeared on the screen again for three seconds. Then, each student could decide to drop a word by clicking on "study again later" or "remove from stack." After the ten-minute study phase, there was a five-minute distraction task during which students had to identify famous people based on photographs. After that, a test was carried out, presenting the Swahili words in random order and asking students to type in the correct English words. Results showed that most students decided to drop a word as soon as they had typed it into the computer correctly once. Results also showed that this was not such a good idea, because recalling a word correctly at least twice improved the score on the test by 26 percent.

This is a good example of how learners can benefit from a computerized program that does the scheduling for them. It keeps track of which words have been acquired already and which ones need to be repeated. With those hundreds of words we need to acquire in a short period of time, efficiency is a key factor.

8 Word Analysis

Word Categories

We have analyzed the rehearsal and matching process when creating a record of a word, and now we can go into further detail by differentiating this process in relation to the word category. A general distinction is made between content and function words. Overall, not much research has been carried out to analyze the effect of word categories when acquiring words in another language. Recently, I have conducted a series of experiments to tackle that issue, and some of these are described in this chapter.

When children learn languages at the age of two, they are able to use prepositions such as "in," "under," or "on" to express relations between objects, states, and events. Objects, states, and events are expressed using nouns, verbs, and adjectives. For example, a child might say "car" for everything that moves, or "I sleep" when tired, or "wet" when in the bathtub. Nouns, verbs, and adjectives, and some adverbs, are content words. At the same time, children use prepositions that belong to the category of function words along with conjunctions, fillers, articles, and some adverbs. As Milton (2009) points out, adverbs are difficult to classify. He argues that, depending on the type of adverb, it can be in either category. Of course, around the age of two, children do not use words correctly. For example, they overextend the meaning of nouns and verbs. The morphological encoding is not yet developed and it generally takes another couple of years until content words are used correctly. Function words, however, are not as overextended as content words and they lack bound or system morphemes that need to be attached. Therefore, it is possible that content and function words are processed differently.

Distinguishing between function and content words is important in the everyday learning of a second language. Content and function words differ in the frequency of their occurrence (Aitchison, 2003; Milton, 2009). Content words are seemingly unlimited in number whereas the number of function words is quite small. The same function words occur more often in any given written or spoken text, because they bind content words into a meaningful sentence. Aitchison (2003) described this process as follows: function words are the glue that holds the sentence together and content words being the bricks, with each brick carrying an independent meaning. Naturally, this implies that function words do not have an independent meaning.

On average, a second language learner enrolled in a second language class is asked to acquire about fifty words per week, as outlined in most textbooks. At the beginner's level, three quarters of those will be content words. Later, at the intermediate level, there will be even fewer function words to learn. Only about one of every ten new words will be a function word. As Schmitt (2010a) pointed out, second language learners often report having difficulties with function words. These problems occur at every level of proficiency. As beginners, there is the problem of acquiring function words for the first time. As advanced learners, there is still the challenge of using them accurately. This is a bit of a surprise because, given the limited number of function words, they should not only have been processed to long-term memory but also recalled with accuracy. A good example is the use of prepositions. In German, grammatical rules dictate which prepositions use the direct object, the indirect object, or indicate a relationship between objects. However, the meaning of the preposition varies and can often not be directly translated from English. The English preposition "for" is most often used in German in the sense of "bei" [at], "nach" [to; in relation to things], or "zu" [to; in relation to living things], but not in the sense of "für" [for]. A common mistake among native English speakers who are learners of German at all levels of proficiency is an overuse of "für." These learners have difficulties finding the correct meaning of the preposition in context, which in turn determines which grammatical rule applies.

This example illustrates the problem during recall, since matching the phonemes to the lexeme of the function word is influenced by the rehearsal process of the content words that the preposition is used with. In Figure 9, the differences between content and function words are exemplified by showing a comparison between a verb and a conjunction. The verb carries more information because the lexeme can be used to combine it with another lexeme (compounds). Verbs also have bound or system morphemes that feed information back to the lexeme and can be used in different tenses by changing the form. Conjunctions do not have any of these characteristics. The discrimination process of content words is therefore more complex than for function words, since there is more to process. The problem with processing function words is that there is not much to discriminate them against. It is almost an either/or situation. Either the function word is processed right away or it is not. In contrast, content words might take more time to be rehearsed in the phonological loop, but all the information they come with assists in the rehearsal process.

Moreover, in concurrence with Aitchison's (2003) argument regarding independent meaning, the lexeme of a content word expresses a rich concept via the lemma, whereas the lexeme of a function word does not. The process of

	phonemes	lexeme/compounds	morphemes	graphemes	other info	word type
to run	[' rʌn]	run/runaway	-s -ing	r-u-n	ran – run (irregular)	verb
laufen	[' laufn]	lauf/Laufweg	-e/-st/-t/-en	l-a-u-f-e-n	lief - gelaufen (irregular)	verb
because	[bɪ ' kɒz]	because	-	b-e-c-a-u-s-e	-	conjunction
weil	[vail]	weil	-	w-e-i-l	-	conjunction

Figure 9. Content vs. Function Words.

matching phonemes to lexemes in function words resembles the binding of phonemes to lexemes in non-words. Non-word repetition relies heavily on processing phonemes, since they do not have existing lexemes. Therefore, a new lexeme needs to be created when rehearsing a non-word, which makes it difficult to bind the phonemes to the lexeme. Both cases rely on temporary storage in the loop, which buys time to identify the phonemes. This tends to be challenging for the learner. Relying on the temporary storage of the loop means that the non-word or function word needs to be rehearsed quite often. When we encounter a function word for the first time, we might need to repeat it more often than a content word in order for it to be processed to long-term memory. At least, that is the hypothesis.

A report regarding the differences between content and function words came from Trojano, Stanzione, and Grossi (1992). They studied a thirty-three-year-old Italian male who, while in his mid-twenties, was admitted to the hospital with sudden memory loss. It was determined that the memory loss was caused by severe aphasia to the left temporal and parietal regions. The temporal region is particularly important for language comprehension (Wernicke's area is in the left temporal region), as well as memory. The information is fed to the mesial region, where the hippocampus creates a record of the word. The auditory cortex and the amygdala both pass through the temporal lobe. The patient, called S. C. in the literature, had to relearn words. In a pre-test on verbal repetition, it was determined that he was able to repeat words but not non-words. The study then continued and distinguished between content words (concrete and abstract nouns) and function words. The patient had to recall those words after they were presented verbally and visually. Results showed that he did much better recalling the visually presented words compared to the spoken words. When presented verbally, he made several mistakes regarding the order of words to be recalled (words were presented in sets of three at a time). He also made more mistakes trying to recall function words than he did with content words.

Another study was conducted around the same time by Neville, Mills, and Lawson (1992). It utilized the EEG technique that measured signals passing through the brain by attaching electrodes to the scalp. The researchers presented adult native English speakers with English sentences consisting of six to thirteen words. The sentences, presented visually on a monitor, were constructed so that the last word would determine if the sentences made sense or not. For example, "Each April we must pay our income tax" vs. "The winning candidate was preparing his acceptance wood." Participants had to determine whether or not the sentence was correct by pressing a button. They did very well, scoring between 98 percent and 100 percent. What was important was that the sentences were presented one word at a time with 700 milliseconds between them. When hearing a natural sentence, a pause of 700 milliseconds represents a substantial amount of time, since we speak at a rate of two words per second. In this study, each word was presented visually and the EEG measured the onset of each word, which is the moment the processing starts after the word was heard. It also measured the duration of processing each word and which brain region was active during that process. A problem with EEG is a time delay between the point of measurement at the scalp and the point of the activity inside the brain. However, the signal strength for both content and function words was measurable. It turned out that, when hearing a function word, the onset was up to 70 milliseconds earlier than it is when hearing a content word. The duration of processing depended on word length. However, when measuring words of equal length, content words were processed slightly longer than function words (between 50 and 100 milliseconds). It seems logical that content words start being processed (onset) a little later after they are heard, because the lemma has to be recognized. It also seems logical that identifying a morphological marker does take a few milliseconds, so the duration of processing is a bit longer. With regard to the brain regions, the EEG showed that for function as well as content words, parts of the prefrontal cortex, parietal lobe, and temporal lobe were active. However, for content words the parietal lobe was activated on the left and right hemisphere of the brain, and for the function words it was mostly activated on the left side only.

Why was the right side not activated when function words were processed? Words were presented one by one to form a sentence. The right side of the parietal lobe is important for feeding visual information from the occipital lobe to the hippocampus. It seems that participants did not register the function words as much as the content words because they were waiting for the next content word to give meaning to the sentence.

It is possible that the right side of the parietal lobe was activated but not enough to show up on the EEG. However, in an article that summarizes these types of studies, Pulvermüller (1999) links this research to his own on the perisylvian cortex. The perisylvian cortex is an ensemble of brain regions in the left hemisphere, including Broca's and Wernicke's areas. Pulvermüller argues that, although content and function words are both processed in the perisylvian cortex, the cortices that transmit information from content words to and from the hippocampus have bilateral links in both hemispheres of the brain, whereas the cortices of function words mostly go through the left hemisphere. In a response to his article, which was published in the journal *Behavioral and Brain Sciences*, several researchers criticized the fact that a lot of the details still have to be worked out when it comes to word processing, although most of them agreed that processing words is very complex and depends on many factors. Therefore, it is possible that words of different categories, such as function words, might indeed be processed differently.

Testing Content and Function Words

In the following paragraphs, we will focus on the general distinction of content vs. function words in second language acquisition. Between 2011 and 2013, I conducted three studies to investigate if second language learners truly have difficulties acquiring function words at the beginner's level.

The first experiment (Schütze, 2015) was carried out with seventy-six undergraduate students enrolled in a beginner's German class at a West Coast university in North America. Students had to fill out a questionnaire to determine their eligibility for the study; for example, they were not allowed to have previous knowledge of German. Students were divided into two groups. One group of students learned content and function words using a uniform interval and the other group using an expanded interval. All students watched a PowerPoint that presented content and function words by giving the English word first (on the left side of the slide) and then, after a two-second delay, the German word (on the right side of the slide) was shown for six seconds. The English word remained on the slide while the German word was shown. Each German word came with audio that was recorded and pronounced by a native speaker as an MP3 file, which was integrated into each PowerPoint slide. Participants had to copy down the German word on a piece of paper after they saw and heard it. For the group following a uniform spacing schedule, the PowerPoint was shown a total of four times in a two – three – two interval (two-day break – three-day break – two-day break). Ideally, a uniform schedule is 100 percent uniform, for example, as a two – two – two interval. However, the class schedule did not permit that. For the group following an expanded interval, the PowerPoint was also shown four times, but in a zero – one – three interval (next day – one-day break – three-day break). The number of four practice sessions was based on previous experiments (Schütze and Weimer-Stuckmann, 2011), which showed that a minimum of four encounters (initial encounter plus three repetitions) was needed in this type of learning situation to process words into long-term memory. Each PowerPoint presented twenty-four content words, which were subdivided into eight nouns, eight verbs, and eight adjectives, as well as fifteen function words, which were subdivided into five prepositions, five conjunctions, and five adverbs. The order of the words was random and different in each PowerPoint, to avoid testing effects. Word selection was based on two criteria. The first criterion was "frequency" and, by using Jones and Tschirner's dictionary (2006), we could ensure that the words were common words. The second criterion was to avoid any interference with the beginner's German class. No words that occurred in the textbook of that class were used. After the practice sessions, participants completed three tests. The first test took place thirty minutes after the last practice (with several distraction tasks in between). The second test was four weeks after the last practice and the third test was eight weeks after. All three tests followed the same format, testing twelve content words and nine function words by presenting the English words visually and asking students to write down the German equivalents. The reason behind not testing all the words was to avoid guessing.

The analysis, using inferential statistics, showed that in both groups students recalled content words more successfully than function words in all of the tests. This difference was statistically significant. It confirmed the hypothesis that function words needed to be rehearsed more often. Regarding the intervals, on the test 1 (short-term gains), the group using the expanded interval scored slightly higher than the group following the uniform interval. However, on test 3 (long-term memory), it was the other way around. The uniform interval group outperformed the expanded interval group. In statistical terms, the difference between the two intervals was not significant.

Compared to the experiments my graduate student and I had carried out using a computerized vocabulary trainer (Schütze and Weimer-Stuckmann, 2011), the overall recall rates in the experiments using PowerPoint slides were lower for both intervals. Using the online trainer, students recalled around 90 percent of the words for both short-term gains and long-term memory, except in the test that was administered months later. In the experiments distinguishing between content and function words, students recalled less than 50 percent on short-term gains and then dropped further on long-term memory. The feedback of the vocabulary trainer had more of an effect than anticipated. If a word was practiced incorrectly, the trainer informed the learner immediately and gave him or her the chance to review the word again.

The results led to more questions. Could we raise the recall rates of content and function words by increasing the number of repetitions to five (as had been done in one set of experiments with the vocabulary trainer (Schütze and Weimer-Stuckmann, 2011)? In that scenario, would the expanded interval still work slightly better for short-term gains and the uniform interval slightly better for long-term memory? Or would we need to reduce the number of words practiced to ease the burden on the phonological loop, Wernicke's area, and the hippocampus?

I carried out two more experiments. In the first of those (the results are published in the same article as the previous experiment on content and function words: Schütze, 2015), I kept the word number at thirty-nine (twenty-four content words and fifteen function words) but increased the interval from four encounters to five encounters. The results confirmed those of the previous experiment: the recall rates for content words were significantly higher than for function words. The extra encounter benefited the learners. All average scores for content and function words were higher compared to the study with one less repetition. The recall rates increased by up to 10 percent. In particular, participants of the expanded group benefitted. They not only had high scores on test 1 (thirty minutes after the last practice session) but also higher scores than the uniform group on test 2 (four weeks after the last practice session). However, the scores dropped in test 3, which was eight weeks after the last practice session. In that test, recall rates for function words were particularly low. In test 3, participants of the uniform group once again had the highest scores. Consistent with the previous experiment, the differences between the two intervals were not significant in statistical terms.

I then conducted a third experiment to test fewer words (twelve content words instead of twenty-four, and nine function words instead of fifteen) and to balance the ratio of content to function words better. This was done to find out if encountering thirty-nine words at once (in each PowerPoint) had been a bit too much for the cognitive load to handle. Students encountered the words five times, as they had in the second experiment. Again, three tests were administered, confirming the results of the first and second study that students recalled content words significantly more than function words. In the test on short-term gains, students using the expanded interval outperformed students using the uniform interval. On the long-term memory test, students using the uniform interval outperformed students using the expanded interval. However, both of these findings were not statistically significant. Furthermore, the rate of recall did not increase, despite the fact that students had to process fewer words.

In summary, the experiments showed that to some extent the expanded interval seemed to benefit students on short-term gains and the uniform interval benefited in the long-term. Using either interval, function words needed to be repeated more often than content words in order to create a record. Also, reducing the number of words is not effective. The phonological loop seemed to be able to handle processing thirty-nine words in a short period of time as long as each word gets the same amount of time to be processed. It seemed to be beneficial to increase the number of repetitions in order to prevent forgetting, which is when, after a couple of months, students would only recall a fraction of the words they had previously learned. The experiments that increased the number of repetitions from four to five showed rising retention rates. A possible explanation lies in the phonological loop itself. Baddeley (2007) proposed that the loop consists of two subsystems: a rehearsal and a temporary storage. The rehearsal is part of Broca's area in the left prefrontal cortex and the temporary storage is in the left side of the parietal lobe. If there is not enough time to process a word right away, it can be stowed in the temporary storage. Reducing the number of words, however, seemed to have no impact on recall rates. This indicates that the interplay of the temporary storage with the rehearsal is more relevant than the sheer number of words to be processed. That being said, there is still naturally an upper limit to the number of words the loop can handle at one time. Therefore, a good strategy for a language learner to improve their retention rate is to increase the number of repetitions. For second language instructors, it might not be the best option to assign less vocabulary to students based on the incorrect premise that the brain cannot handle large amounts of words at once.

As mentioned in Chapter 7, "Spacing," it should be noted that these experiments were conducted in a university setting, where undergraduate students studied German for the first time with no previous knowledge of a second language. Therefore, it should not be concluded that practicing words five times is a magic number for second language vocabulary learning. It proved to be a number that worked in the context described. If any of the variables were changed, the results could have been different – for example, if the learners had a higher proficiency level or if they were in a learning environment where German (or any other language) was predominantly spoken. For languages with a different system of sounds, such as Japanese, Korean, Cantonese or Mandarin, the process of rehearsal will likely have to be repeated many times, as the main task for a learner is to identify phonemes and match them to lexemes.

The results from the three experiments on content and function words were analyzed further by differentiating between word groups. The recall of content words was analyzed with regard to length and similarity. It showed that, out of all the content words tested, longer words and phonologically similar words were recalled the least. However, since the number of words used from these groups in the experiments was fairly low, an analysis using inferential statistics could not be carried out. Still, there is some indication that processing these types of words is difficult when acquiring another language; something that Baddeley (1966a, 1966b; Baddeley, Thomson, and Buchanan, 1975) found several decades ago when conducting experiments in first-language studies.

In the following section, we will learn more about these word groups as well as about words with an emotional connotation.

Word Groups

In Chapter 4, "Cognitive Load," we learned that factors such as word length, phonological similarity, and emotional connotation influence the time it takes to form a record of a new word. These factors are important for content words, because those words can be either short or long, are almost unlimited in number, sometimes similar-sounding, and may have emotional connotations. With regard to function words, these factors play less of a role because they are usually short, limited in number, rarely similar, and lack emotional connotations.

The word length effect showed that longer words are more difficult to process if they cannot be broken down into compounds. It is also important to note that breaking down words into compounds may help, but not always. Longer words are difficult, because there are so many phonemes to process that their memory trace might expire before all of them have been identified. The phonological similarity effect showed that discriminating among similar phonemes also takes time and can lead to mistakes. The effect disappears if words are repeated several times. Words with an emotional connotation are processed with heightened activation. If they are associated with a particular situation or event, the effect is even stronger. It has not yet been established whether it is possible for these words only to need to processing once to create a record. We will discuss this in more detail in the next section.

When learning another language, content words of that language can also be short, long, similar, and/or have an emotional connotation.

An interesting thing about word length is compounding; that is, is when two words are combined into one long word. Each compound has its own lexeme. The degree of compounding depends on the language you are learning. German, for example, is full of compounds that combine nouns, verbs, and adjectives in various ways to make words that get longer and longer. Take the example of "Gepäckausgabe," meaning "luggage claim," from Chapter 4, "Cognitive Load," when we were once again at Frankfurt airport. "Gepäck" means "luggage" and "Ausgabe" means "distribution." You can add the word "Stelle," meaning "place," to that compound to indicate the actual location where you would pick it up. If you are looking for your bike or skis, you will see a sign saying "Sondergepäckausgabestelle," with "sonder" meaning "special." That is the place where you would pick up your special luggage. If you need to talk to someone about that, you need to find the "Sondergepäckausgabestellenpersonal," with "Personal" meaning the people who deal with all issues related to this. Note that, in that case, an "n" was added to "Stelle," which is a feature of some nouns in German. A game sometimes played in a German kindergarten revolves around who can make the longest word.

A useful strategy is to break compound words apart and process the parts. However, some words are simply long without compounds. The actual processing of these words functions the same as it does in a person's first language. In both cases, we face the challenge of running out of time before we have processed all the phonemes and lexeme(s) of a longer word.

When learning another language, similarity can have a positive effect if the word being learned is similar in form and/or meaning to a word in the first language. In this case, it is processed faster because the lexeme already exists in our memory. Those words are called cognates or near cognates. Take the example of "Kaffee" again. You can guess that it means "coffee" just by hearing it pronounced. You will have to make slight adjustments to the lemma because the concept of a "Kaffee" is slightly different than that of a coffee, but overall the lexeme is similar. You will also have to adjust your pronunciation, as some of the phonemes are pronounced differently. Nevertheless, a word like that is processed faster, even though it still depends a bit on the level of proficiency. If you are a beginner and are just starting to learn new words in another language, your memory is happy to recognize anything similar and will process the word quickly. At that level, the slightly different concept of "Kaffee" is acknowledged, but the lexeme is not necessarily adjusted right away. That comes later. If you are at an intermediate level, those adjustments will play more of a role, since you want the record of "Kaffee" to be as accurate as possible. Making those adjustments might take more time and might affect the recall of the word. If you are beginning to learn German and at the airport in Frankfurt using your dictionary to order a coffee, it is likely you will just say "Kaffee." If you are an intermediate learner, you might hesitate a bit. When recalling the word "Kaffee," you wonder if there is another word for "coffee" in German, since by now you know that the lexeme of "Kaffee" is slightly different than that of "coffee." At a higher level of proficiency, usually those differences are accepted by the speaker. You realize that there is a small difference between "Kaffee" and coffee, but "Kaffee" is indeed the word you need to say in this particular situation.

Something you have to be aware of at all levels of proficiency is that some words look similar but have a different meaning. Those are called false friends. A common example of this is the German word "Brand," which does not indicate a brand name but actually means a fire that is burning out of control. Something else to be aware of is the multiple meaning of words. A good example is the German word "Geist," which is similar to the English word "ghost." However, it can also mean "mind," "intellect," or "spirit." A beginner might be happy to simply accept the one meaning "ghost" while a more advanced learner will probably try to process the word correctly with all of its unique meanings. That takes more time, and in that case similarities might not be helpful, because you will think of "ghost" first and the other meanings second. A proficient speaker actually tries to keep words of different languages apart. This has been observed by Singleton (1995, 2007), who also pointed out the individual differences between learners. Some learners will want to process every word correctly with all of its unique features right from the start, whereas others are happy to make compromises. This behavior of an individual learner can be linked to his or her previous knowledge of the L1, as well as to his or her knowledge of any other languages.

In Chapter 4, "Cognitive Load," we learned that in first and second language acquisition similarity of phonemes can have a negative effect on word processing, because it takes longer to distinguish the phonemes. When recalling a word, the string of tags and nodes that are brought up and determine serial order are susceptible to errors. If English is your first language, trying to remember lists of words such as "cat, map, man, hat" would be difficult due to the similarity of the sounds (Baddeley, 1966a, 1966b). In second language acquisition, the same effect comes into play. The phonemes need more time to be discriminated because otherwise some overlap might occur. Learning many new words that sound similar at the same time is never a good idea, as the example of "Reihe" [line/row] and "Reise" [journey/travel] demonstrated. The only difference between the two is the second syllable "h" vs. "s." However, the small difference in the phoneme changes the lexeme entirely. Processing a word to long-term memory, we need to establish the form-to-meaning relationship by matching phonemes to lexemes. If one phoneme changes the lexeme, the likelihood of a processing error increases. Either the word is processed incompletely, incorrectly or it takes more time. The record of the word is weak and it will be difficult to recall it. What we can do is to repeat the word many times; eventually "h" or "s" will be discriminated sufficiently and recorded correctly. What we can also do is to add a word to a word we already know, but it should be one step at a time. For example, if we have already learned "gehen" [ˈgeːən] [to go], we can add "stehen" [ˈʃteːən] [to stand]. The only difference in sound between those two words in German is in the first syllable [g] vs. [ʃt]. We can add words that have a similar lexeme but are phonologically different, such as "kriechen" [ˈkriːçn] [to crawl], "wandern" [ˈvandɐn] [to hike], and "laufen" [ˈlaufn] [to run], although we also have to be careful and try not to acquire too many words with similar lexemes at once.

What has been said about the lexemes of false friends (see the example of "Brand") can also be said, to some degree, about the phonemes. Most phonemes are pronounced differently from language to language. A word in German such as "Wind" looks very similar to the English word "wind" and has an identical meaning. In this case, it is processed very quickly because the lexeme and phonemes seem identical. In reality, while the lexeme is identical, the initial phoneme is not: the German "w" is pronounced like the English "v." Again, individual differences and the proficiency level might determine if the German "Wind" is pronounced correctly. Therefore, the similarity of phonemes might speed up the process of recalling words, but also it might not.

Emotional Activation

We know that emotional words are processed with heightened activation. In this case, the senses are activated releasing more serotonin, dopamine, or acetylcholine into the brain, which in turn either forms or modifies a synapse. Moreover, emotional words are often associated with a particular situation or event. However, when recalling a word, the mechanism of rehearsing phonemes and matching them to a lexeme is the same for all words, whether they are emotional or not. What the heightened activation does is create a strong record that assists in recalling the word at a later point in time. One has to be aware that, when learning another language, heightened activation does not always have a positive effect when recalling a word. For example, it can cause some hesitation.

As stated, our brain recalls lexemes from the non-mesial region, but with each recall they must again undergo the process of discrimination (Mueller et al., 2003). The record of the word created when the word was first processed assists in this process of discrimination. Lexemes are part of the record of a word as well as a tag that indicates the acceptable combination of phonemes to the lexeme. The record also includes information on spelling and non-linguistic information. Phonemes are called up from Wernicke's area, and then they are rehearsed in the loop and matched to lexemes in the loop of Broca's area. A strong record – that is, a rich lexeme or a strong tag or powerful sensual information – speeds up the process of recall, whereas a weak record does not. If the record is too weak, then our brain will not be able to recall the word, or it will only be recalled with additional assistance. That assistance could come when the speaker remembers the situation in which s/he encountered the word, in which case the hippocampus is contacted to see how the record was created. In some cases, remembering another word that was recorded as part of that situation can also help to bring forward the word one is trying to recall, but this requires additional cognitive resources because, in addition to all the phonemes and lexemes that have already been activated, now the phonemes and lexemes linked to second word must also be activated. As these phonemes and lexemes all compete against each other, the discrimination process will take more time. There is also the possibility that a word may be temporarily unavailable because the tag is not activated enough. The delay can be caused due to the nature of the record, as a weak record does not assist in the process of discrimination. There can also be a delay if the opposite happens – that is, if the record of the word is very strong – in particular if an emotional word needs to be expressed. If an emotional word was encountered in a particular situation, then sensory information about the time and place of that situation may have been recorded along with the linguistic information. In order to recall that word in a different situation, the hippocampus might be consulted on whether the word can be used in that new situation. This all takes some time to decide, and helps to explain why it is at times difficult to express ourselves with emotional words.

Apart from individual preferences of the speaker, a key factor in this process is the level of proficiency. At a lower level of proficiency, heightened activation leads to faster processing. The emotional word stands out, particularly if it is tied to a situation, because the high dose of the neurotransmitter, paired with the stimulation of the senses and the amygdala, contributes to the record of the word, which is then stored in the non-mesial region. From this, a new synapse is created. The word should be recalled with relative ease, because recalling the record of an emotional word as part of a situation is tied to this array of non-linguistic information. Coming back to the example of "heiß" [hot] when drinking a coffee at Frankfurt airport, the sensation of burning your tongue is part of the record. If the word "heiß" was encountered without the experience of burning your tongue, there is still heightened activation, since it is a sensory word. However, the activation is not as strong as in combination with the actual experience of burning your tongue. At a higher level of proficiency, most learners are aware that emotional words in L1 and L2 do not always share the same concepts. Although the emotional word is processed quickly, there could be some hesitation when using it, due to a slightly different concept. A good example is the German word "Angst." We mentioned this word in Chapter 2, "Memory, Language, and the Brain." A highly proficient speaker knows that the word "Angst" does not only equal "fear" but rather it is a mixture of "anxiety" and "fear." It can also be compounded; for example, "Existenzangst" expresses the feared anticipation of losing all possessions, either materialistic or spiritual. If the speaker is searching their memory to find a word that suits "Angst" better, that search would be hindered, because the heightened activation of the word "Angst" makes it more difficult to activate other words. If this is paired with an event, the hesitation would be even greater. Unfortunately, there is not a word in English that equals "Angst" and searching for an equivalent expends resources until that is realized. Of course, a simple solution is to code switch and say "Angst."

Regarding word concepts, Altarriba, Bauer, and Benvenuto (1999) carried out an interesting study with monolingual speakers of English, comparing concrete, abstract, and emotional words. The speakers were given a word and had to write down the first word that came to mind that was meaningfully related to the given word. All in all, 55 speakers were given 352 words each: 100 concrete words (for example, "car"), 154 abstract words (for example, "liberty"), and 98 emotional words (for example, "joy"). Results showed that the words written down for the emotional words produced the highest number of different associates. That is a good indication of how multifaceted the concept of an emotional word is. Now imagine learning another language, such as German, where all the emotional words also have multifaceted concepts. Understanding those concepts and expressing them by choosing the right word will be a difficult task indeed. Initially, a learner can imitate. In fact, this is what children do when they start learning a language. Eventually, though, relationships between the words and concepts need to be formed, which is when processing becomes more difficult. Coming back to the example of the "Kaffee" and burning your tongue in Frankfurt airport, imagine you stay in Germany for a while and become proficient. Eventually, someone asks you about your first experience in Germany and you tell him or her the story of the coffee. In German, of course. Then, after some time, you go back to North America and want to tell the same story in English. It will be difficult, because you remember the story in German with words that were tied to an event in Germany.

One question we still have not answered is whether we need to bother repeating emotional words when we encounter them, or if they so overpowering that they are immediately processed to long-term memory. Is it possible that a record in the form of a synapse is created the first time an emotional word is encountered?

In an experiment I conducted in 2015, I presented twenty-four words to three groups of students. Group 1 saw each word once; group 2, three times; and group 3, five times. There were twenty-four students in group 1, twenty-seven students in group 2, and twenty-five students in group 3. Twelve of those words had an emotional connotation (four nouns, four verbs, four adjectives) and the other twelve (four nouns, four verbs, four adjectives) did not. Students were enrolled in "Beginning German I" courses at a West Coast university in North America and spoke English as their first language. The words were presented one at a time in a PowerPoint presentation, with the English word shown first for two seconds, followed by the German word for six seconds while the English word remained on the screen. Each German word came with audio that was recorded and pronounced by a native speaker as an MP3 file that had been integrated into each PowerPoint slide. The order of the words was changed for each viewing to avoid testing effects. Students viewed the PowerPoint at the beginning of class. The words selected were not from the textbook of the course. Groups 2 and 3 viewed the words more than once and followed the expanded interval due to practical considerations. The course met Tuesdays, Wednesdays, and Fridays resembling a zero – one interval (group 2: three encounters: Tuesday, Wednesday, Friday), and a zero – one – three – six interval (group 3: five encounters: Tuesday, Wednesday, Friday, Tuesday, following Tuesday).

Two tests were carried out. Test 1 took place at the end of class, which was thirty minutes after the last encounter of the words. The distraction included a grammar lecture and grammar activities in between. Test 2 occurred four weeks after that.

Results showed that participants in five of the six tests (three groups: two tests per group) recalled more emotional words than non-emotional words (except for test 1 of group 2, where participants recalled more non-emotional words). None of the differences were statistically significant. In fact, differences in recall rates were minimal throughout. For both, emotional and non-emotional words, participants in group 3 (five encounters) recalled more words than participants in group 2 (three encounters), who recalled more words than participants in group 1 (one encounter). Recall rates were similar to those of previous studies (Schütze, 2015).

The answer to our research question – Is a record of an emotional word created the first time it is encountered? – is that it is unlikely. Some participants in group 1 recalled one or two emotional words in the third test, but they also recalled one or two non-emotional words in that test. In order to attain higher recall rates, it is as beneficial to repeat emotional words as it is to repeat non-emotional words. Why were emotional words not fast-tracked? A possible explanation is that the sensory information that is fed through the cortices to the hippocampus when processing words to long-term memory (Gluck and Myers, 2001; Milner, Squire, and Kandel, 1998; Amaral et al., 1992) was not heightened enough to create a higher dose of a neurotransmitter. Watching and listening to words on a PowerPoint was not enough stimulation to produce higher levels of serotonin, dopamine, or acetylcholine. In order to heighten the senses, an actual emotional situation needs to be created. Remember when you burned your tongue drinking "heißer Kaffee" at Frankfurt airport? The senses were heightened and that information became part of the record of the word "heiß."

A follow-up question asks how much sensual information would be needed; for example, if the words presented in the PowerPoint would be accompanied by images. It has been shown that providing visual information improves the recall rates of words in second language vocabulary learning (Jones and Plass, 2002; Kim and Gilman, 2008; Rimrott, 2010). We can assume that, if images had been added to the PowerPoint slides in the experiment presented here, recall rates would probably have gone up. However, the question is whether they would have gone up more for emotional than non-emotional words. An experiment investigating this issue is being planned.

The experiment comparing recall rates of emotional and non-emotional words was subject to a second analysis I carried out that distinguished between female and male participants. In Chapter 3, "Synaptic Connections," we asked whether women and men process emotional words differently. The rationale is that estrogen levels in women are higher than in men, which is important, because estrogen is able to stimulate serotonin. Therefore, women might have an advantage when processing emotional words.

The ratio of female to male students in each group was well balanced. Of the twenty-four students in group 1, twelve were female and twelve male; of the twenty-seven students in group 2, fifteen were female and twelve male; and of the twenty-five students in group 3, twelve were female and thirteen male. Results showed that the recall rates in each group were similar for female and male students on all tests. Both – female and male students – recalled significantly fewer words in test 2 (four-week delayed post-test) compared to test 1 (immediate post-test thirty minutes after rehearsal) measured using inferential statistics (ANOVA).

In summary, in the context of acquiring a second language at a college or university in North America, five rehearsals seem necessary to attain high recall rates regardless of the student population (female vs. male students) and whether or not words have an emotional connotation. However, more studies in this area are needed to verify the results. It would be interesting to carry out experiments focusing on five repetitions. Several research agendas could be pursued: one, to compare more emotional and non-emotional words than just twelve each; two, to enhance words with images to investigate if that has more of an impact on words with an emotional connotation or words with no emotional connotation; and three, to increase the number of female and male students.

In conclusion, does this mean we should create an emotional situation when learning a new word, even if the word itself is not emotional? In theory, the emotional situation would be fast-tracked. The situation is part of the record that is created. When the word needs to be recalled from the non-mesial region, two things occur: first, lexemes are brought up and rehearsed; and second, if needed, the non-linguistic information that was recorded is also brought up. Therefore in theory, learning a non-emotional word by creating an emotional situation might speed up the process of creating a record of that word. However, there are some issues with that type of approach, and we will return to those issues in the final chapter of this book.

9 Learning and Teaching

Efficient Acquisition and Recall

Throughout this book, we have learned that the process of recording a new word depends on several factors:

- the situation (modalities: audio, visual, example)
- the word group (length, similarity, emotional connotation)
- the word category (content vs. function words)
- the spacing (uniform vs. expanded)
- the timing (number of repetitions, time frame).

As research has shown, in order to create a record of a word it needs to be repeated. In order to store the record of a word permanently, even though nothing is permanent when it comes to forming synapses, it seems that repeating a word using a uniform interval is most beneficial. However, for short-term gains, using an expanded interval might be the better option. The number of repetitions is linked to the learning environment. In this book, we have focused on acquiring new words as adult learners in an environment where the language to be learned is not predominantly spoken. In that environment, a general guideline is to repeat a word four times using a "one plus four" (initial encounter plus four repetitions) design for a total of five practice sessions. These practices should take place over a time period of two weeks, and each time elaborative processing should be used. Elaborate processing takes place when the word is not just recognized but actively produced. Regarding the word category and word groups, function words need more repetition than content words. Longer and phonologically similar words also need time to be rehearsed and must be repeated often. In contrast, words with an emotional connotation that were encountered in an emotional situation can be fast-tracked into long-term memory. The more the senses are involved when encountering a word, the more it assists with creating a record of that word.

The purpose of acquiring new words in another language is to communicate meaningfully with another person who speaks that language. This can be done face-to-face as well as through Skype, chat, email, text, or a written note, all of which requires the person to be able to actively use words in that language. Those words need to be recalled from memory, which activates the non-mesial region, the phonological loop, Broca's area, Wernicke's area, and, if needed, the hippocampus. This is a matter of processing speed: it has to be done in seconds or less. In fact, when speaking an entire sentence, we use half a second or less per word. So how should we study for this?

Before we discussing this, we need to remember the three components of speech: fluency (speed of recalling the words from memory), accuracy (correct recall of those words including grammatical coding), and complexity (having many records of words stored including those that have multiple meanings). These three components depend on the situation in which the word is acquired, the word itself, the level of proficiency of the speaker, the phase of development, and his or her background, as well as preferences, which include the motivation and the willingness to make compromises.

What also factors into any language learning is the accumulation of new experiences that influence the fluency, accuracy, and complexity of the speech. More and more information can be added to a lemma. Once a lemma has been formed and becomes part of a lexeme, it also holds some grammatical information as to how the concept is applied in different contexts. The lexeme can be expanded by refining the lemma, which expresses the concept of the word and how it is used. This can happen when a word is encountered a second time. Every time we encounter a word it is processed, and every time we recall a word it is processed again. When a word is processed, the phonemes and lexemes are discriminated, identified, and strengthened. Part of that process can include encoding new information to the lemma.

Studies on attention (Robinson, 2003; Skehan, 1998, 2009a) have shown that our capacity to process information is limited. If a word is recalled quickly by finding the correct combination of phonemes to the lexeme, it still might not be recalled accurately, due either to problems with the morphemes or whether it is a complex lexeme. In particular, learners who have just begun acquiring another language often have to make a choice between using a word incorrectly and not using it at all. What we learned from studies on attention is that we cannot overburden the cognitive load. Less is more. In fact, reducing the amount of material to be remembered is one of several strategies that Gathercole and Alloway (2008) outline in their book on working memory and learning. However, the cognitive load can handle more than we sometimes assume. For example, in the context of adult second language acquisition at a university or college, we can learn forty words at a time if we space them out using the uniform or expanded interval (Schütze, 2015). What we learned from all the studies conducted on spacing is that, when acquiring a new word, there is no point in repeating it several times in a row. In that scenario, the phonemes and lexemes would not stop being processed. In order for repetition to be effective, the process has to start anew every time a word is repeated. This is done by introducing distractions or by letting time pass in between each repetition. Evidence for that comes from studies on the phonological loop (Baddeley, 2007) and studies on sleep (Raichle, 2011).

When creating a record of a word, neurons begin to fire. They then synchronize their efforts and converge to process the information (Singer, 2006; Tranel and Damasio, 2002). Synapses can be created or modified. A synaptic bridge makes it easier to recall words. We need to keep in mind that, not only linguistic information is processed that way but also non-linguistic information, such as information related to the senses.

In summary, we have learned that the acquisition of words in another language is a multidirectional, dynamic, and fluid process in which information is exchanged constantly, involving language and memory faculties as well as the senses.

How to Learn and How not to Learn New Words

As learners, we sometimes try to overcompensate by repeating a word we need to remember for a vocabulary quiz over and over. Then, when we do the quiz, we cannot remember that word. However, a word comes to mind that we did not constantly repeat. It is similar to playing football (the one you play with your feet) or hockey. If you aim for the post, you rarely hit it. If you aim for the goal, you hit the post all the time. You cannot force the issue.

Attempting to learn new words just before a test, for example, will most likely not be very successful. The reason is simple. In order to learn it, we have to repeat it as well as take breaks in between. If we have not left ourselves much time before a test, we may choose to rehearse the word several times without taking a break. This is known as massed learning, which results in an automatic processing stage where, the second and third time we rehearse a word, the word does not receive the attention it needs because it is still being processed in the loop. If the attention goes down, activation of the language faculties also goes down. Less activity leads to less processing and, therefore, the phonemes and lexemes are not discriminated sufficiently. Consequently, it will be more difficult to recall that word.

What we can do is to make sure we learn smarter and review the words we need to acquire efficiently. This requires studying words within a certain time frame, a certain number of times, and with defined intervals in between.

When learning new words, we have to think about our intentions. If we are looking to acquire words to only be used in the next few days (for example, going on vacation), repeating them five times using an expanded interval can lead to substantial gains. If we want to recall those words months later (for example, for another language course), we might want to use a uniform interval instead. This is supported by the neurophysiology of information processing. If we start off by repeating words in shorter periods of time using an expanded interval, more synaptic connections are built, but they are fragile. It is as though the cement to build the synaptic bridge is not yet dry when the next layer is put on. It is different with the uniform interval, where enough time passes from repetition to repetition for the cement to dry. However, fewer synapses are built, due to the time it takes to wait for the cement to dry. So, while more words are recalled on short gains when an expanded interval is used, more of those words are forgotten in the long run, because the cement was still wet and eventually flushed out. This tendency was shown in second language acquisition studies (Schütze, 2015). In an ideal world, we would do both. We would start by practicing the words five times with the expanded interval and then continue to repeat the words once a week using a uniform interval for maintenance. The problem is that most of us do not have time for that. But, coming from the perspective of how words are processed in the brain, it makes perfect sense.

We also have to think about how many words we can learn at a time. As pointed out previously, the cognitive load is robust but there is still a limit to how much we can take in. In the context of learning words in a country where the language to be learned is not the one that is predominantly spoken, we can probably acquire forty words in a time period of two weeks if they are properly spaced (Schütze, 2015). Of course, the actual number varies from individual to individual, since other factors, such as motivation, knowledge of other languages, and proficiency level, play a role. Something that should be avoided when learning words for a test is attempting to learn too many words in too little time, such as the day before. This is referred to as cramming and is bound to fail. What can work is refreshing one's memory the day before a test. For example, you have just forgotten the meaning of a word and look it up again in a dictionary. If you had learned this word before, looking it up might help to strengthen the record that was created and, therefore, if it comes up on a test, you might have a good chance of recalling it successfully. The same scenario applies in a situation where you know you are going to need certain words – for example, when ordering "ein Kaffee" in Germany. You already learned this word but, to be sure, you look it up one more time before going to the coffee stand.

We now know that emotional words are fast-tracked if they are associated with a situation or event. A question we asked earlier in this book is if we should create an emotional situation to acquire non-emotional words. Although this seems like a good idea in theory, there are three issues to consider.

The first issue is practical. It is difficult to create an emotional situation for every word we learn. The second issue has to do with classical conditioning. Remember how the sea slug *Aplysia* started to remember its reflex to withdraw the gill after repeatedly being stimulated? Any organism will adapt over time. If all words are learned emotionally, the fast-tracking advantage will be lost, because it will become the norm. The third issue has to do with attention. We need to direct attention to an incoming word but that happens only if it is considered necessary to the executive control function in the brain. Attention is limited; therefore the executive control is constantly weighing whether it deserves our attention or not. In a way, we would have to trick the executive control into focusing its attention on an artificial learning situation.

Creating an artificial learning situation has failed before. The language labs of the 1970s are proof of that (Korte, 2009). These labs were built to try to provide a communicative situation where learners could practice certain phrases. When sitting in a language lab, the brain is asking why you are talking to a machine and not a person. Nowadays, the technology has improved, using animations, computer-generated voices, or avatars. Yet, the brain is asking the same question. Some online language programs use a real person in a video that you can click on. However, there is still no natural interaction. A video we click on has been pre-programmed. The person in the video can ask you questions and can even recognize your answers as correct or incorrect but only if you give an answer that was one of the pre-programmed responses. However, try asking the person in the video a question that has not been pre-programmed. The executive control in our brain will recognize this as an artificial conversation and will soon divert attention to something more interesting, such as picking up the phone and actually talking to someone. As in the 1970s, someone who uses such a program today would find that, when visiting the country of the language s/he is trying to learn, s/he could say very little. This person might understand quite a bit, but the production skills are underdeveloped, such as having trouble being able to speak fluently with few mistakes and stringing words together in meaningful sentences. That does not imply that technology cannot be used to support the learning of another language. We just have to acknowledge its limitations and focus on the things that it can do for us. For example, we can use algorithms to program spacing intervals into an online tool that will assist us in the process of acquiring new words. Furthermore, the research on word groups and word categories suggests it is important to differentiate between the different types of words based on their length, similarity, emotional connotation, and whether they are content words or function words. The results from these studies imply that it would be a mistake to treat all words the same and ignore these factors. Unfortunately, word learning programs and textbooks seem to pay little attention to what is going on in our brain, particularly under what conditions words are processed to long-term memory. For example, if function words need many rehearsals, those words should be treated differently when learning another language.

How we process words relies on our knowledge of words that we have already acquired as well as how we use that knowledge. A record of a word needs to be created before making associations with other new words. Using word fields or word trees, which are often used in textbooks, is making the process of discriminating phonemes and lexemes more difficult. It overburdens the capacity of the loop. Using a word tree or field is only useful if the number of words to be acquired is small and some of the words in the field or tree are known already.

If we acquire words via a word tree or word field, a problem known as associative blocking might occur. This means that the record of one word is stronger than the record of another word. The stronger word can therefore suppress the activation of the other words even if it is the one you are trying to recall (Anderson, Bjork, and Bjork, 1994).

A classic study comes from Barnes and Underwood (1959), who asked students to remember a list of nonsense syllables that were paired with adjectives. They then had students remember another list with the same nonsense syllables, except this time they were paired with different adjectives. On a test carried out twenty-four hours after the learning phase, students had to recall the adjective when prompted by the nonsense syllable. Some students were given the second list once. Others were given the second list five times, ten times, or twenty times. Results showed that when the first and the second lists were studied once each, significantly more adjectives were recalled correctly from the first list, because the pair on the first list suppressed the pair on the second list. This can be explained by the fact that a record of the first pair was created before the second pair was encountered. Creating a record for the second pair is more difficult, because it has to compete with a word that has just been processed. Therefore, the second list needs to be studied several times.

What should always be avoided is to learn words that are phonological similar all at once. A sequence such as "gehen – stehen – geben – nehmen – sehen – leben" [go/walk – stand – give – take – see – live] will likely be very difficult to recall, since in German each word sounds very similar to one another [ˈge:ən – ˈʃte:ən – ˈge:bn – ˈne:mən – ˈze:ən – ˈle:bn]. We might recall the sounds, but not the meaning of each of those words. In fact, if a list like that is used and some time later we hear the word "gehen," those other words might come to mind, but we might have no idea what they mean in English. What we can do is break the sequence up into pairs – for example, "gehen – stehen" [go/walk – stand] – which is better, since there are now only two items and they are related in meaning. Another example would be "geben – nehmen" [give – take].

A sequence of words works better with lexemes if they are not similar-sounding, such as "gehen – kriechen – wandern – laufen" [ˈge:ən – ˈkri:çn – ˈvandɐn – ˈlaufn] [go/walk – crawl – hike – run]. However, it is not recommended to create a sequence that is too long. If done in moderation, we can create phrases with a word; for example, "nach Hause gehen," "in die Schule gehen," and "zum Fußballspiel gehen" [go home, go to school, and go to a football match]. At the same time, this will help to practice the use of function words such as the prepositions "nach" [to], "in" [in, to], and "zum = zu dem" [to]. A word such as "Fußball" can be extended by adding other words to it; for example, "Fußballspiel," "Fußballschuhe," and "Fußballverein" [football match, football shoes, football club]. Again, one has to be careful not to create words that are too long.

With regard to pronunciation, a good strategy is to learn the sounds of a new language correctly right from the beginning. To do this, it is important to learn how the letters of the alphabet are pronounced, including diphthongs. Diphthongs are combinations of vowels such as [ou] in English. Remember the example that I gave on British English on the words "though," "through," and "plough" in Chapter 1, "A New Word"? Even though all of these use the same diphthong, [ou], some of them are pronounced differently. "Though" is pronounced how the diphthong [ou] is pronounced in most words. However, "through" and "plough" are different and therefore require more attention, which costs energy. Having practiced the diphthong [ou] and its variations helps learners of English as a second language to process words that are exempt from the regular pronunciation of [ou]. Fortunately, not all languages have this many variations in pronunciation. Nevertheless, even for a language such as German, which has fairly simple rules regarding pronunciation, practicing the pronunciation of the alphabet, including diphthongs, will assist when processing a new word.

Smart Systems

The next question is how the process of acquiring many new words can be optimized when learning another language in high school, college, university, or on your own. After all, there are thousands of words to be learned. Although most European languages have a repertoire of more than 100,000 words, knowing 5,000 words will give a student the ability to communicate effectively by either speaking or writing (Schmitt, 2010b), because 5,000 words represent about 85 percent of the words used in everyday interaction. This can be accomplished by learning eight words per day. In the context of teaching a foreign language at college or university, many textbooks are structured so that students learn only 2,500 words in the first two years. Still, as some researchers report, it is surprising how little vocabulary students can remember after a two-year language program at university (Milton, 2009). Many of the words that have been learned from the textbook are forgotten quickly.

In his model of what it means to know a word, Nation (2001) distinguishes between form (spoken/written) and meaning (concepts/relationships). The questions he raises are how form and meaning interact, what parts of a word are needed in order to recognize or produce a word, and what other words the word is associated with. Furthermore, some aspects of how words are used in multiple contexts also play a role.

While the form-to-meaning relationship needs to be established right from the start when acquiring new words, the other aspects of form, meaning, and multiple usages should not be neglected. Unfortunately, this is how most textbooks operate. Analyzing the vocabulary presented and practiced in four German textbooks published in North America and used for first-year German courses at college or university in the United States and Canada, Neary-Sundquist (2015) found that these textbooks almost exclusively focus on the form-to-meaning relationship.

Another problem with textbooks is that they do not usually recycle words very well. For example, if words are introduced in one chapter, they are not necessarily used again in subsequent chapters (Tschichold, 2012). In addition, little attention is paid to repeating words at the point of introduction (Nation, 2009; Zimmerman, 2009).

Tschichold (2012) analyzed a French textbook for learners of English and found that many words are presented in an unstructured format and that it is left up to the learner and/or teacher to make sense of it all. López-Jiménez (2010) analyzed twenty-four textbooks teaching Spanish and English. She pointed out that in English textbooks vocabulary is often recycled too much and in Spanish textbooks it is recycled too little. In general, considerations of repetition, frequency, or cognitive load are ignored. A classic example is that some words that are in glosses next to a text are not even in the text. Similarly, online environments such as *Second Life* provide little assistance to the learner (Milton et al., 2012).

A popular way to learn words is to use flashcards. The idea of flashcards first sprung up in the 1960s. At the time, linguists were becoming more and more interested in how language is processed in the brain; however, the focus was on grammar. After some flashcard memory systems were developed, these systems found their way into schools but were not researched any further. Some of these systems were still used well into the 1990s and into this century. The recent discoveries in neurophysiology on how memories are formed have once again sparked interest in the cognitive processing of language. Much of that interest is now directed toward word acquisition.

Flashcards have the advantage of providing information using several modalities, which caters to different learning styles (Kim and Gilman, 2008; Oxford, 2003; Rimrott, 2010).

Zimmermann (2009) recommended that, when using flashcards on paper, a computer, or a smartphone, one should add information every time a word is used, but at the same time she cautions not to write too much information on the cards because this could cause confusion. We also know that it will overload cognitive capacity. As to what type of information should be on the card, Zimmerman recommended the meaning of the word, as well as examples of how that word is used. We also know that pictures are helpful, as they stimulate the senses to process non-linguistic information. Overall, the learner should have the option to decide how much of that information s/he wants to see at the same time or in succession (Nation, 2001). Furthermore, learners need to be given the opportunity to produce a word (Barcroft, 2015; Webb, 2005).

If we think about the development of flashcard systems in terms of Star Trek, the order would be: flashcard systems on paper (such as "Die Lernkartei" by Leitner in 1972 – the Original), flashcards on a computer (such as by Mondria and Mondria-De Vries in 1994 – the Next Generation), and flashcard programs that provide smart feedback to the learner (Voyager). A good question is how much research actually goes into the development of these so-called smart flashcards or systems.

In our research (Schütze and Weimer-Stuckmann, 2011) where we developed a vocabulary trainer (Schütze and Weimer-Stuckmann, 2010), we asked what type of intervals are most beneficial in spacing practices. We also distinguished between short-term gains and long-term retention. A few years later, I asked how many words the cognitive load can handle at a time and differentiated between word categories and groups (Schütze, 2015).

Based on this research, my graduate student and I developed the vocabulary trainer further. The trainer – ViVo© (Virtual Vocabulary), and ViVoSmart© (the app version) – takes into consideration the complexity of processing words into long-term memory, including: the interplay of rehearsing phonemes to lexemes in the phonological loop, finding the correct combination with help from Wernicke's area, identifying morphemes, and adding non-linguistic information via the hippocampus and sometimes the amygdala. Using the trainer, learners can choose from various spacing intervals. Each word is presented with several modalities (picture, audio, translation, sample sentences, and grammar info), as illustrated in Figure 10. The modalities highlighted in white can be viewed at once, and the ones highlighted in black are hidden behind the icon in order not to overload the amount of information a learner has to digest. It is up to the learner to read the sample sentences and/or get grammatical information. Likewise, when learners are asked to recall the words they have learned, they are only presented with a picture, but have the option to get additional information when clicking on the "Sample Sentences" (where the target word is left blank) and "Grammar Info" icons.

A key feature of the trainer is that learners are asked to practice words actively by typing out each word (where it says "blank"). The trainer provides immediate feedback by underlining the word in green or red, depending on whether or not it was typed out correctly. In addition, the trainer keeps track

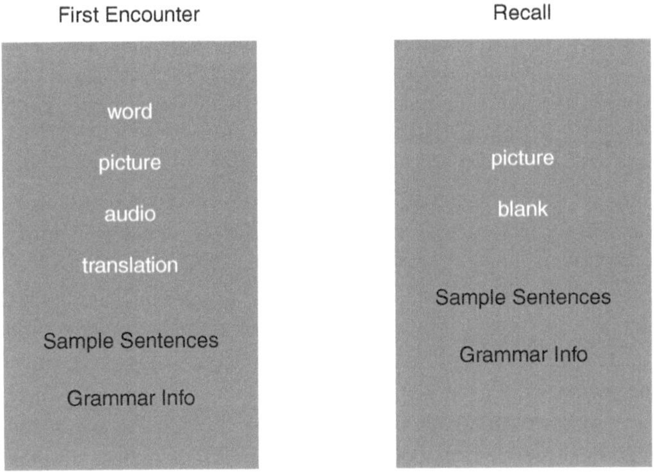

Figure 10. ViVoSmart©.

on the words which have been acquired as well as those which need to be repeated. When logging on, the trainer suggests to the learner which words should be practiced at that time. In theory, it helps the learner to acquire words efficiently.

What Now?

The theme of this book is how words are processed in the brain. We have learned that the acquisition of words varies from learner to learner. Individual factors such as the phase of development, knowledge of one's first or other languages, motivation, skills, and preferences all play a role. So does the environment we are acquiring the language in. We have also learned about proficiency levels, in particular that when reaching a higher proficiency level some of the individual factors might have changed. Throughout the book, we focused on situations that apply to many of us attempting to learn another language as adults.

We also briefly touched on what happens when we learn a language as a child, as well as what happens when we get into our sixties and beyond.

When learning a language, the optimal learning experience for children is similar to that of adults. Strictly speaking, both need comprehensible and complex input. Language learning means developing speech that is fluent, accurate, and complex. While for children this is a first-time experience, adults can rely on having gone through that process before. The speech of parents as well as language instructors needs to be fluent, accurate, and complex, because they are the main source from which children and adults usually acquire their language skills. At the same time, the cognitive load should not be overburdened. Therefore, giving long monologues might not be the best idea, because that will provide too much information to process. Instead, the conversation should be interactive, giving the child and the adult learner a chance to practice the words that they have just heard. For younger children as well as adults, the ability to repeat non-words is important in order to process words. Both older children and adults use the knowledge of words they already know to identify new words.

Naturally, there are some differences between children learning a language compared to adults. Adults are already familiar with language as a system and can therefore acquire grammatical rules faster. When acquiring words, however, the tables are turned. Children acquire thousands of words quickly once the vocabulary explosion sets in around the age of two. For adults, the speed of acquiring thousands of new words depends largely on the situation, and the factors that I have outlined above.

What happens when a child is exposed to two languages? In this case, it is ideal if the child receives fluent, accurate, and complex input in both languages. There also has to be a sufficient amount of input. If the caregivers have different first languages, each should interact with the child in their respective first languages, because the vocabulary is most likely more rich in the first language than the second. Similarly, the pronunciation and grammatical coding is likely more fluent, accurate, and complex in the first language as well. If both caregivers speak the same first language but live with their child in a country where another language is predominantly spoken, it is advisable to keep speaking to the child in that first language so the child continues to receive the necessary input. What is important in this situation is that the child also speaks in their first language to other children who speak that language. A child can learn how to play with the language from other children, for example, by making up words such as a "crayon stripe" to mean "rainbow." That is part of the learning process. At the same time, the child needs input from children and adults who speak the language that is predominant in the country that they are living in. This is usually provided when a child goes to school.

When learning another language, we have to keep in mind that there are five sensitive phases that mark the development of our language acquisition. We need to build connections between phonemes and lexemes (until six to eight years of age), develop strategies (around eight), analyze abstractions (eleven to fourteen), develop the loop (six to sixteen), and create memories (six to twenty-five). Ideally, we learn and practice another language during all of these phases, the last of which is in our mid-twenties, when the workings of the phonological loop, Wernicke's area, Broca's area, and the hippocampus are optimized.

Building connections and creating memories continues throughout life. However, somewhere in our mid-sixties, our memory starts to slowly decline, impacting our ability to recall words. The chemicals in our body change. For example, the production of the neurotransmitters serotonin, dopamine, and acetylcholine slows down (Scheibel, 1992). Starting around that age, not all synapses continue to receive the proper maintenance. Synapses begin to dissipate and words are forgotten. This is a normal process. Can we still learn another language when we are older? Actually, we can. It just takes more time. When acquiring new words, they need to be repeated many times and ideally in a setting where non-linguistic information can also be recorded; for example, when traveling to another country. The concept of intrinsic motivation (Deci and Ryan, 1985, 2002) is particularly important. It is the feeling of being engaged in the process of learning for personal reasons, as opposed to being forced to learn.

In conclusion, when encountering new words in another language the pressure is on remembering as many words as possible in a short period of time in order to successfully communicate in that language. However, research conducted in the neurosciences, cognitive psychology, and second language acquisition suggests that a bit of patience might go a long way. By this, I am referring to repeating the new words several times and making sure there is a sufficient break between each repetition. The hippocampus needs some time to create a record of a word. The second repetition should occur after the first one has been forgotten, because then the process of recording the word starts over again. Each new recording stimulates the record until the lexeme, the combination of phonemes, and other sensory information are stored in the non-mesial region. A synapse is created or modified to allow permanent access, although that synapse still has to be maintained. It seems that spacing the repetitions in an expanded interval works well for short-term gains, and repeating words using a uniform interval works well for committing words to long-term memory. However, other factors, such as the proficiency level, motivation, and the situation in which the word is acquired, all play a role. The number of repetitions is linked to the word category and group. In particular, emotional words that are part of a situation or event can play a special role, as can function words. It is a good idea to try to learn words by imitating; for example, by listening to the pronunciations and speaking them out loud. If possible, it would also be beneficial to associate a word with an image. Finally, when encountering and acquiring new words in another language, we have to be careful not to overload the phonological loop by processing too many words at a time. In short, we need to do ourselves a favor and give our memory a chance to keep up.

Bibliography

Abrahams, J. P., and Camp, C. J. (1993). Maintenance and generalization of object naming training in anomia associated with degenerative dementia. *Clinical Gerontologist*, 12(3), 57–72.

Aitchison, J. (1992). Slip of the Tongue. In T. McArthur (ed.), *The Oxford Companion to the English Language* (p. 114). Oxford University Press.

(2003). *Words in the Mind: An Introduction to the Mental Lexicon.* Oxford: Blackwell.

Aleman, A. (2013). *Wenn das Gehirn älter wird. [When the Brain Ages.]* Munich: Beck.

Alloway, T. P. (2006). How does working memory work in the classroom? *Educational Research and Reviews*, 1(4), 134–39.

Allport, A., Styles, E. A., and Hsieh, S. (1994). Shifting attentional set: exploring the dynamic control of tasks. In C. Umilta and M. Moscovitch (eds.), *Attention and Performance,* vol. 15, *Conscious and Nonconscious Information Processing* (pp. 421–62). Cambridge, MA: MIT Press.

Altarriba, J., Bauer, L., and Benvenuto, C. (1999). Concreteness, context-availability, and imageability ratings and word associations for abstract, concrete, and emotion words. *Behavior Research Methods, Instruments, and Computers*, 31, 578–602.

Altarriba, J., and Isurin, L. (eds.) (2013). *Memory, Language and Bilingualism.* Cambridge University Press.

Amaral, D., Prince, J., Pitkanen, A., and Carmichael, S. (1992). Anatomical organization of the primate amygdaloid complex. In J. P. Aggleton (ed.), *The Amygdala: Neurobiological Aspects of Emotion, Memory, and Mental Dysfunction* (pp. 1–66). New York: Wiley.

Anderson, M. C., Bjork, R. A., and Bjork, E. L. (1994). Remembering can cause forgetting: retrieval dynamics in long-term memory. *Journal of Experimental Psychology: Learning, Memory and Cognition*, 20, 1063–87.

Archibald, J. (1998). *Second Language Phonology.* Amsterdam: John Benjamins.

Archibald, L. M. D., and Gathercole, S. E. (2006). Short-term and working memory in specific language impairment. *International Journal of Language & Communication Disorders*, 41(6), 675–93.

(2007). Nonword repetition and serial recall: equivalent measures of verbal short-term memory? *Applied Psycholinguistics*, 28, 587–606.

Awh, E., Jonides, J., Smith, E. E., Schumacher, E. H., Koeppe, R. A., and Katz, S. (1996). Dissociation of storage and rehearsal in verbal working memory: evidence from positron emission tomography. *Psychological Science*, 7, 25–31.

Baddeley, A. D. (1966a). Short-term memory for word sequences as a function of acoustic, semantic and formal similarity. *Quarterly Journal of Experimental Psychology*, 18, 362–65.

(1966b). The influence of acoustic and semantic similarity on long-term memory for word sequences. *Quarterly Journal of Experimental Psychology*, 18, 302–09.

(1966c). The capacity of generating information by randomization. *Quarterly Journal of Experimental Psychology*, 18, 119–29.

(1986). *Working Memory*. Oxford University Press.

(1999). *Essentials of Human Memory*. Hove: Psychology Press.

(2007). *Working Memory, Thought, and Action*. Oxford University Press.

Baddeley, A. D., Eysenck, M. W., and Anderson, M. C. (2009). *Memory*. Oxford: Psychology Press.

Baddeley, A. D., Gathercole, S. E., and Papagno, C. (1998). The phonological loop as language learning device. *Psychological Review*, 105, 158–73.

Baddeley, A. D., and Hitch, G. (1974). Working memory. In G. H. Bower (ed.), *The Psychology of Learning and Motivation: Advances in Research and Theory* (vol. 8, pp. 47–89). New York: Academic Press.

Baddeley, A. D., Papagno, C., and Vallar, G. (1988). When long-term learning depends on short-term storage. *Journal of Memory and Language*, 27, 586–95.

Baddeley, A. D., Thomson, N., and Buchanan, M. (1975). Word length and the structure of short-term memory. *Journal of Verbal Learning and Verbal Behaviour*, 14, 575–89.

Balota, D., Duchek, J., and Logan, J. (2007). Is expanded retrieval practice a superior form of spaced retrieval? A critical review of the extant literature. In J. Nairne (ed.), *The Foundations of Remembering: Essays in Honor of Henry L. Roediger* (vol. 3, pp. 83–105). New York: Psychology Press.

Balota, D. A., Duchek, J. M., Sergent-Marshall, S. D., and Roediger, H. L. (2006). Does expanded retrieval produce benefits over equal-interval spacing? Explorations of spacing effects inh aging and early stage Alzheimer's disease. *Psychology and Aging*, 21(1), 19–31.

Barcroft, J. (2004). Effects of sentence writing in second language lexical acquisition. *Second Language Research*, 20(4), 303–34.

(2015). Can retrieval opportunities increase vocabulary learning during reading? *Foreign Language Annals*, 48(2), 236–49.

Barnes, J. M., and Underwood, B. (1959). "Fate" of first-list associations in transfer theory. *Journal of Experimental Psychology*, 58, 97–105.

Basso, A. H., Spinnler, G., Vallar. G., and Zanobio, E. (1982). Left hemisphere damage and selective impairment of auditory verbal short-term memory: a case study. *Neuropsychologica*, 20, 263–74.

Bauer, P. J. (2004). Getting explicit memory off the ground: steps toward construction of a neuro-developmental account of changes in the first two years of life. *Developmental Review*, 24, 347–73.

Bloom, I., and La Heij, W. (2003). Semantic facilitation and semantic interference in word translation: implications for models of lexical access in language production. *Journal of Memory and Language*, 48, 468–88.

Bishop, D., Adams, C., and Norbury, C. (2004). Using nonword repetition to distinguish genetic and environmental influences on early literacy development: a study of 6-year-old twins. *American Journal of Medical Genetics*, 129B, 94–96.

Buchsbaum, B. R., and D'Esposito, M. (2008). The search for the phonological store: from loop to convolution. *Journal of Cognitive Neuroscience*, 20(5), 762–78.

Burgess, N., and Hitch, G. J. (1999). Memory for serial order: a network model of the phonological loop and its timing. *Psychological Review*, 106, 551–81.

Carpenter, S. K., and DeLosh, E. L. (2005). Application of the testing and spacing effects to name learning. *Applied Cognitive Psychology*, 19, 619–36.

Cenoz, J., Hufeisen, B., and Jessner, U. (eds.) (2003). *The Multilingual Lexicon*. Dordrecht: Kluwer.

Chen, L., Shu, H., Liu, Y., Zhao, J., and Li, P. (2007). ERP signatures of subject-verb agreement in L2 learning. *Bilingualism: Language and Cognition*, 10(2, 161–74.

Cheung, H. (1996). Non-word span as a unique predictor of second language vocabulary learning. *Developmental Psychology*, 32(5), 867–73.

Clark, E. V. (1973). What's in a word? On the child's acquisition of semantics in his first language. In T. E. Moore (ed.), *Cognitive Development and the Acquisition of Language* (pp. 65–110). New York: Academic Press.

Cohen, J. D., Perlstein, W. M., Braver, T. S., Nystrom, L. E., Noll, D. C., Jonides, J., and Smith, E. E. (1997). Temporal dynamics of brain activation during a working memory task. *Nature*, 386, 604–07.

Cook, V., and Singleton, D. (2014). *Key Topics in Second Language Acquisition*. Clevedon: Multilingual Matters.

Cowan, N. (1992). Verbal memory span and the timing of spoken recall. *Journal of Memory and Language*, 31, 668–84.

(1993). Activation, attention, and short-term memory. *Memory & Cognition*, 21(2), 162–67.

(1999). An embedded-processes model of working memory. In A. Miyaki and P. Shah (eds.), *Models of Working Memory: Mechanisms of Active Maintenance and Executive Control* (pp. 62–101). Cambridge University Press.

Craik, F., and Lockhart, R. S. (1972). Levels of processing: a framework for memory research. *Journal of Verbal Learning and Verbal Behaviour*, 11, 671–84.

Cull, W. (2000). Untangling the benefits of multiple study opportunities and repeated testing for cued recall. *Applied Cognitive Psychology*, 14(3), 215–35.

Davidson, M., Amso, D., Aderson, L. C., and Diamond, A. (2006). Development of cognitive control and executive functions from 4 to 13 years: evidence from manipulations of memory, inhibition, and task switching. *Neuropsychologia*, 44(11), 2037–78.

de Bot, K. (1992). A bilingual production model: Levelt's "speaking" model adapted. *Applied Linguistics*, 13, 1–24.

(2004). The multilingual lexicon: modelling selection and control. *International Journal of Multilingualism*, 1, 17–32.

de Bot, K., Lowie, W., and Verspoor, M. (2007). A Dynamic Systems Theory approach to second language acquisition. *Bilingualism: Language and Cognition* 10(1), 7–21.

de Bot, K., and Schreuder, R. (1993). Word production and the bilingual lexicon. In R. Schreuder and B. Weltens (eds.), *The Bilingual Lexicon* (pp. 191–214). Amsterdam: John Benjamins.

Deci, E. L., and Ryan, R. M. (1985). *Intrinsic Motivation and Self-Determination in Human Behavior*. New York: Plenum.

(eds.) (2002). *Handbook of Self-Determination Research.* Rochester: University of Rochester Press.

De Groot, A. M. B. (1992). *Bilingual Lexical Representation: A Closer Look at Conceptual Representations.* In R. Frost and L. Katz (eds.), *Orthography, Phonology, Morphology, and Meaning* (pp. 389–412). Amsterdam: Elsevier Science Publishers.

(2006). Effects of stimulus characteristics and background music on foreign language vocabulary learning and forgetting. *Language Learning*, 56(3), 463–506.

DeLange, R. J., Kemp, R. G., Riley, W. D., Cooper, R. A., and Krebs. E. (1968). Activation of skeletal muscle phosphorylase kinase by adenosine triphosphate and adenosine 3', 5'-monophosphate. *Journal of Biological Chemistry*, 243(9), 2200–08.

Dell, G. S. (1988). The retrieval of phonological forms in production: tests of predictions from a connectionist model. *Journal of Memory and Language*, 27, 124–42.

Dell, G. S., and Reich, P. (1981). Stages in sentence production: an analysis of speech error data. *Journal of Verbal Learning and Verbal Behavior* 20(6), 611–29.

Diamond, A. (2002). Normal development of prefrontal cortex from birth to young: adulthood cognitive functions, anatomy, and biochemistry. In D. T. Stuss and R. T. Knight (eds.), *Principles of Frontal Lobe Function* (pp. 466–503). New York: Oxford University Press.

Diamond, A., and Taylor, C. (1996). Development of an aspect of executive control: development of the abilities to remember what I said and to "Do as I say, not as I do." *Developmental Psychobiology*, 29(4), 315–34.

Dijkstra, T., and Van Heuven, W. (1998). The BIA model and bilingual word recognition. In J. Grainger and A. M. Jacobs (eds.), *Localist Connectionist Approaches to Human Cognition* (pp. 189–225). Mahwah, NJ: Erlbaum.

(2002). The architecture of the bilingual word recognition system: from identification to decision. *Bilingualism: Language and Cognition*, 5, 191–98.

Doughty, C. J. (2003). Instructed SLA: constraints, compensation, and enhancement. In C. J. Doughty and M. L. Long (eds.). *The Handbook of Second Language Acquisition* (pp. 256–310). Oxford: Blackwell.

Draaisma, D. (2004). *Why Life Speeds Up as You Get Older.* Cambridge University Press.

Ebbinghaus, H. (1913). *Grundzüge der Psychologie. [Fundamentals of Psychology.]* Leipzig: Viet.

Ellis, N. (1996). Phonological memory, chunking, and points of order. *Studies in Second Language Acquisition*, 18, 91–126.

Fell, J., Klaver, P., Lehnertz, K., Grunwald, T., Schaller, C., Elger, C., and Fernández, G., (2001). Human memory formation is accompanied by rhinal-hippocampal coupling and decoupling. *Nature Neuroscience*, 4(12), 1259–64.

French, L., and O'Brien, I. (2008). Phonological memory and children's second language grammar learning. *Applied Psycholinguistics*, 29(3), 463–87.

Fromkin, V. (1973). Slips of the tongue. In V. Fromkin (ed.), *Speech Errors as Linguistic Evidence.* The Hague: Mouton.

Furnham A., and Bradley, A. (1997). Music while you work: the differential distraction of background music on the cognitive test performance of introverts and extraverts. *Applied Cognitive Psychology*, 11, 445–55.

Garagnani, M., Wennekers, T., and Pulvermüller, F. (2006). A neuronal model of the language cortex. *Neurocomputing*, 70, 1914–19.

Gathercole, S. E., and Alloway, T. P. (2008). *Working Memory and Learning: A Practical Guide for Teachers*. London: Sage Publications.

Gathercole, S. E., and Baddeley, A. D. (1989). Evaluation of the role of phonological STM in the development of vocabulary in children: a longitudinal study. *Journal of Memory and Language*, 28, 200–13.

(1990). Phonological memory deficits in language-disordered children: is there a causal connection? *Journal of Memory and Language*, 29, 336–60.

Gathercole, S. E., Pickering, S. J., Ambridge, B., and Wearing, H. (2004). The structure of working memory from 4 to 15 years of age. *Developmental Psychology*, 40, 177–90.

Gathercole, S. E., Pickering, S. J., Hall, M., and Peaker, S. (2001). Dissociable lexical and phonological influences on serial recognition and serial recall. *Quarterly Journal of Experimental Psychology*, 54A, 1–30.

Gergely, Z. (2007). Selection of grammatical morphemes in early bilingual development. In Z. Lengyel and J. Navracsics (eds.), *Second Language Lexical Process* (pp. 133–45). Clevedon: Multilingual Matters.

Gleason, J. B. (ed.) (2001). *The Development of Language*. Boston: Pearson, Allyn and Bacon.

Gluck, M., and Myers, C. (2001). *Gateway to Memory: An Introduction to Neural Network Modeling of the Hippocampus in Learning and Memory*. Cambridge, MA: MIT Press.

Green, D. W. (1986). Control, activation, and resource. *Brain and Language*, 27, 210–23.

Grosjean, F., and Li, P. (2013). *The Psycholinguistics of Bilingualism*. Chichester: Wiley-Blackwell.

Hasselhorn, M. (2005). Lernpotential Arbeitsgedächtnis. Wie verändert es sich him Verlauf der menschlichen Lebensphase? [Learner potential working memory. How does it change during the course of human life spans?] In Akademie der Wissenchaften zu Göttingen (ed.), *Jahrbuch der Akademie der Wissenchaften zu Göttingen* (pp. 302–07). Göttingen: Vandenhoeck and Ruprecht.

Hebb, D. O. (1949). *The Organization of Behavior*. New York: Wiley.

(1961). Distinctive features of learning in the higher animal. In J. F. Delafresnaye (ed.), *Brain Mechanisms and Learning* (pp. 37–46). Oxford: Blackwell.

Herculano-Houzel, S. (2009). The human brain in numbers: a linearly scaled-up primate brain. *Frontiers Human Neuroscience*, 3, 31.

Hulstijn, J. H. (2001). Intentional and incidental second-language vocabulary learning: a reappraisal of elaboration, rehearsal and automaticity. In P. Robinson (ed.), *Cognition and Second Language Instruction* (pp. 258–86). Cambridge University Press.

Hulstijn, J. H., and Laufer, B. (2001). Some empirical evidence for the involvement load hypothesis in vocabulary acquisition. *Language Learning*, 51(3), 539–58.

Indefrey, P., and Levelt, W. J. M. (2004). The spatial and temporal signatures of word production components. *Cognition*, 92, 101–44.

Ittner, L. M., Ke, Y., Delerue, F., Bi, M., Gladbach, A., van Eersel, J. Wölfing, H., Chieng, B., Christie, M., Napier, I., Eckert, A., Staufenbiel, M., Hardeman, E., and Götz, J. (2010). Dendritic function of tau mediates amyloid-beta toxicity in Alzheimer's disease mouse models. *Cell*, 142(3), 387–97.

Jacobs, B. (1988). Neurobiological differentiation of primary and secondary language acquisition. *Studies in Second Language Acquisition*, 10, 303–37.

Jiang, N. (2000). Lexical representation and development in a second language. *Applied Linguistics*, 21(1), 47–77.

Jones, L. C., and Plass, J. L. (2002). Supporting listening comprehension and vocabulary acquisition in French with multimedia annotations. *Modern Language Journal*, 86(4), 546–61.

Jones, R. L., and Tschirner, E. (2006). *A Frequency Dictionary of German*. London: Routledge.

Kandel, E. R. (2006). *In Search of Memory. The Emergence of a New Science of Mind*. New York: W. W. Norton & Co.

Kim, D., and Gilman, D. (2008). Effects of text, audio, and graphic aids in multimedia instruction for vocabulary learning. *Educational Technology and Society*, 11(3), 114–26.

Kim, K. H., Relkin, N. R., Lee, K.-M., and Hirsch, J. (1997). Distinct cortical areas associated with native and second languages. *Nature*, 388, 171–74.

Koenigs, M., Acheson, D., Barbey, A., Solomon, J., Postle, B., and Grafman, J. (2011). Areas of left perisylvian cortex mediate auditory-verbal short-term memory. *Neuropsychologia*, 49, 3612–19.

Kornell, N., and Bjork, R. A. (2010). Optimising self-regulated study: the benefits – and costs – of dropping flashcards. *Memory*, 16(2), 125–36.

Korte, M. (2009). *Wie Kinder heute lernen. [How Children Learn Today.]* Munich: Deutsche Verlags-Anstalt.

Krebs, E. G., DeLange, R. J., Kemp, R. G., and Riley, W. D. (1966). Activation of skeletal muscle phosphorylase. *Pharmacology Review*, 18, 163–71.

Kroll, J. F., and Dijkstra, T. (2010). The bilingual lexicon. In R. B. Kaplan (ed.), *The Oxford Handbook of Applied Linguistics* (pp. 349–72). Oxford University Press.

Kroll, J., Michael, E., Tokowicz, N., and Dufour, R. (2002). The development of lexical fluency in a second language. *Second Language Research*, 18, 137–71.

Kroll, J., and Stewart, E. (1994). Category interference in translation and picture naming: evidence for asymmetric connections between bilingual memory representations. *Journal of Memory and Language*, 33, 149–74.

Kupfermann, I. and Kandel, E. R. (1969) Neuronal controls of behavioral response mediated by the abdominal ganglion of Aplysia. *Science*, 164, 847–50.

Landauer, T., and Bjork, R. (1978). Optimal rehearsal patterns and name learning. In M. Grüneberg, P. Morris, and R. Sykes (eds.), *Practical Aspects of Memory* (pp. 625–32). London: Academic Press.

Larsen-Freeman. D. (1997). Chaos/complexity science and second language acquisition. *Applied Linguistics*, 18, 141–65.

Larsen-Freeman, D., and Cameron, L. (2008). *Complex Systems and Applied Linguistics*. Oxford University Press.

Laufer, B. (1997). What's in a word that makes it hard or easy: some intralexical factors that affect the learning of words. In N. Schmitt and M. McCarthy (eds.), *Vocabulary. Description, Acquisition, and Pedagogy* (pp. 140–55). Cambridge University Press.

Leitner, S. (1972). *So lernt man Lernen: Der Weg zum Erfolg. [Learning to Learn: The Road to Success.]* Freiburg: Herder.

Lenneberg, E. (1967). *Biological Foundations of Language*. New York: Wiley and Sons.

Levelt, W. J. M. (1989). *Speaking: From Intention to Articulation*. Cambridge, MA: MIT Press.

(1992). Accessing words in speech production: stages, processes and representations. *Cognition*, 42, 1–22.

Levelt, W. J. M., Roelofs, A., and Meyer, A. S. (1999). A theory of lexical access in speech production. *Behavioral and Brain Sciences*, 22, 1–75.

Levitin, D. J. (2008). *The World in Six Songs: How the Musical Brain Created Human Nature*. Toronto: Penguin Canada.

Logan, J. M., and Balota, D. A. (2008). Expanded vs. equal interval spaced retrieval practice: exploring different schedules of spacing and retention interval in younger and older adults. *Aging, Neuropsychology, and Cognition*, 15(3), 257–80.

Logie, R. H., Cocchini, G., Della Sala, S., and Baddeley, A. (2004). Is there a specific capacity for dual-task co-ordination? Evidence from Alzheimer's disease. *Neuropsychology*, 18, 504–13.

López-Jiménez, M. D. (2010). The treatment of lexical aspects in commercial textbooks for L2 teaching and learning. In R. Chacón-Beltrán, C. Abello-Contesse, and M. del Mar Torreblance-López (eds.), *Insights into Non-native Vocabulary Teaching and Learning* (pp. 156–74). Bristol: Multilingual Matters.

Mackey, A., Adams, R., Stafford, C., and Winke, P. (2010). Exploring the relationship between modified output and working memory capacity. *Language Learning*, 60(3), 501–33.

Meara, P. (1984). The study of lexis in interlanguage. In A. Daves, C. Criper, and A. Howatt (eds.), *Interlanguage* (pp. 225–39). Edinburgh University Press.

(2009). *Connected Words: Word Associations and Second Language Vocabulary Acquisition*. Amsterdam: John Benjamins.

Merriënboer, J. J. G., and Sweller, J. (2005). Cognitive load theory and complex learning: recent developments and future directions. *Educational Psychology Review*, 17(2), 147–77.

Miller, P. (2002). *Theories of Developmental Psychology*, 4th ed. New York: Worth Publishers.

Milner, B., Squire, L. R., and Kandel, E. R. (1998). Cognitive neuroscience and the study of memory. *Neuron*, 20(3), 445–68.

Milton, J. (2009). *Measuring Second Language Vocabulary Acquisition*. Bristol: Multilingual Matters.

Milton, J., Jonsen, S., Hirst, S., and Lindenburn, S. (2012). Foreign language vocabulary development through activities in an online 3D environment. *Language Learning Journal*, 40(1), 99–112.

Molnár, H. (2010). Der Einfluss des Faktors Alter auf die Aussprachekompetenz in der L2: Ergebnisse einer Pilotstudie mit DaZ-Lernern. [The influence of the factor age on the competence of pronounciation in L2: results of a pilot study with DaZ-learners.] *Zeitschrift für Interkulturellen Fremdsprachenunterricht*, 15(1), 19. Available at http://tujournals.ulb.tu-darmstadt.de/index.php/zif/index

Mondria, J., and Mondria-De Vries, S. (1994). Efficiently memorizing words with the help of word cards and "hand computer": theory and applications. *System*, 22(1), 47–57.

Mueller, S. T., Seymour, T. L., Kieras, D. E., and Meyer, D. E. (2003). Theoretical implications of articulatory duration, phonological similarity, and phonological complexity in verbal working memory. *Journal of Experimental Psychology: Learning, Memory, and Cognition*, 29(6), 1353–80.

Müller, N., and Knight, R. (2006). The functional neuroanatomy of working memory contributions of human brain lesion studies. *Neuroscience*, 139, 51–58.

Murray, D. J. (1968). Articulation and acoustic confusability in short-term memory. *Journal of Experimental Psychology*, 78, 679–84.

Muzur, A., Pace-Schott, E. F., and Hobson, J. A. (2002). The prefrontal cortex in sleep. *Trends in Cognitive Science*, 6(11), 475–81.

Myers-Scotton, C. (2003). Code-switching: evidence for both flexibility and rigidity in language. In J.-M. Dewaele, A. Housen, and Li Wei (eds.), *Bilingualism: Beyond Basic Principles* (pp. 189–203). Clevedon: Multilingual Matters.

Myers-Scotton, C., and Jake, J. (2000). Four types of morpheme: evidence from aphasia, code switching, and second language acquisition. *Linguistics*, 38, 1053–100.

Nagy, N. (1997). Modeling contact-induced language change. *University of Pennsylvania Working Papers in Linguistics*, 25(4), 399–418.

Nation, I. S. P. (2001). *Learning Vocabulary in Another Language*. Cambridge University Press.

(2009). *Teaching Vocabulary: Strategies and Techniques*. Boston: Heinle.

Neary-Sundquist, C. (2015). Aspects of vocabulary knowledge in German textbooks. *Foreign Language Annals*, 48(1), 68–81.

Neville, H. J., Mills, D. M., and Lawson, D. S. (1992). Fractionating language: different neural subsystems with different sensitive periods. *Cerebral Cortex*, 2(3), 244–58.

O'Connor, M., Butters, N., and Miliotis, P. (1992). The dissociation of anterograde and retrograde amnesia in a patient with herpes encephalitis. *Journal of Clinical and Experimental Neuropsychology*, 14, 159–78.

Oxford, R. L. (1990). *Language Learning Strategies: What Every Teacher Should Know*. Boston: Heinle.

(2003). Language learning styles and strategies: concepts and relationships. *International Review of Applied Linguistics in Language Teaching*, 41, 271–78.

Page, M. P. A. and Norris, D. (1998). The primacy model: a new model of immediate serial recall. *Psychological Review*, 105, 761–81.

Papagno, C., Valentine, T., and Baddeley, A. D. (1991). Phonological short-term memory and foreign-language vocabulary learning. *Journal of Memory and Language*, 30, 331–47.

Papagno, C., and Vallar, G. (1992). Verbal short-term memory and the learning of novel words: the effects of phonological similarity and item length. *Quarterly Journal of Experimental Psychology*, 44A, 47–67.

Paradis, M. (1994). Neurolinguistic aspects of implicit and explicit memory: implications for bilingualism and SLA. In N. Ellis (ed.), *Implicit and Explicit Learning of Languages* (pp. 393–419). London: Academic Press.

Pavlenko, A. (2009). Conceptual representation in the bilingual lexicon and second language vocabulary learning. In A. Pavlenko (ed.), *The Bilingual Mental Lexicon. Interdisciplinary Approaches* (pp. 125–60). Clevedon: Multilingual Matters.

Petersen, S. E., Fox, P. T., Posner, M. I., Mintun, M., and Raichle, M. E. (1989). Positron emission tomographic studies of the processing of single words. *Journal of Cognitive Neuroscience*, 1(2), 153–70.

Piaget, J. (1955). *The Construction of Reality in the Child*. New York: Basic Books.

(1962). *The Language and Thought of the Child*. London: Routledge.

Pickering, S. J., and Gathercole, S. E. (2001). *The Working Memory Test Battery for Children*. Oxford: Psychological Corporation.

Pimsleur, P. (1967). A memory schedule. *Modern Language Journal*, 51, 73–75.

Pollock, E., Chandler, P., and Sweller, J. (2002). Assimilating complex information. *Learning and Instruction*, 12, 61–86.

Port, R. (2007). How are words stored in memory? Beyond phones and phonemes. *New Ideas in Psychology*, 25, 143–70.

Postle, B. R. (2006). Working memory as an emergent property of the mind and brain. *Neuroscience*, 139, 23–38.

Pulvermüller, F. (1996). Hebb's concept of cell assemblies and the psychophysiology of word processing. *Psychophysiology*, 33, 317–33.

(1999). Words in the brain's language. *Behavioral and Brain Sciences*, 22, 253–79.

(2000). Cell assemblies, axonal conduction times, and the interpretation of high-frequency dynamics in the EEG and MEG. In R. Miller (ed.), *Time and the Brain* (pp. 241–49). Newark, NJ: Harwood Academic.

Pulvermüller, F., Shtyrov, Y. Ilmoniemi, R., and Marslen-Wilson, W. (2006). Tracking speech comprehension in space and time. *NeuroImage*, 31, 1297–305.

Raichle, M. (2010). Two views of brain function. *Trends in Cognitive Science*, 14(4), 180–90.

(2011). The restless brain. *Brain Connectivity*, 1, 3–12.

Raichle, M., MacLeod, A. M., Snyder, A., Powers, W., Gusnard, D., and Shulman, G. (2001). A default mode of brain function. *Proceedings of the National Academy of Science*, 98(2), 676–82.

Richmond, J. and Nelson, C. A. (2007). Accounting for change in declarative memory: a cognitive neuroscience perspective. *Developmental Review*, 27, 349–73.

Rimrott, A. (2010). Computer-assisted vocabulary learning: multimedia annotations, word concreteness, and individualized instruction. Ph.D. thesis dissertation, Simon Fraser University. Available at http://summit.sfu.ca/item/11876.

Robinson, P. (2003). Attention and memory during SLA. In C. J. Doughty and M. H. Long (eds.), *The Handbook of Second Language Acquisition* (pp. 631–78). Oxford: Blackwell.

Robinson, B., and Mervis. C. (1998). Disentangling early language development: modeling lexical and grammatical acquisition using and extension of case-study methodology. *Developmental Psychology*, 34, 363–75.

Roediger, H. L., and Karpicke, J. D. (2010). Intricacies of spaced retrieval: a resolution. In A. S. Benjamin (ed.), *Successful Remembering and Successful Forgetting: Essays in Honor of Robert A. Bjork* (pp. 1–36). New York: Psychology Press.

Rolke, B., Heil, M., Streb, J., and Henninghausen, E. (2001). Missed prime words within the attentional blink evoke an N400 semantic priming effect. *Psychophysiology*, 38, 165–74.

Rothbart, M. K., and Posner, M. I. (2005). Genes and experience in the development of executive attention and effortful control. In L. A. Jensen and R. W. Larson (eds.), *New Horizons in Developmental Theory and Research* (pp. 101–08). San Francisco: Jossey-Bass.

Routtenberg, A., and Rekart, J. L. (2005). Post-translational protein modification as the substrate for long-lasting memory. *Trends in Neurosciences*, 28(1), 12–19.

Schacter, D. L., Rich, S. A., and Stampp, M. S. (1985). Remediation of memory disorders: experimental evaluation of the spaced-retrieval technique. *Journal of Clinical and Experimental Neuropsychology*, 7(1), 79–96.

Scheibel, A. B. (1992). Structural changes in the aging brain. In J. E. Birren, R. B. Sloane, and G. Cohen (eds.), *Handbook of Mental Health and Aging* (pp. 147–73). New York: Academic Press.

Schmidt, R. (1995). Consciousness and foreign language learning: a tutorial on the role of attention and awareness in learning. In R. Schmidt (ed.). *Attention and Awareness in Foreign Language Learning* (pp. 1–64). Honolulu: University of Hawai'i Press.

(2001). Attention. In P. Robinson (ed.), *Cognition and Second Language Instruction* (pp. 3–32). Cambridge University Press.

Schmitt, N. (2010a). Key issues in teaching and learning vocabulary. In R. Chacón-Beltrán, C. Abello-Contesse, and M. del Mar Torreblance-López (eds.), *Insights into Non-native Vocabulary Teaching and Learning* (pp. 28–40). Clevedon: Multilingual Matters.

(2010b). *Researching Vocabulary*. Basingstoke: Palgrave Macmillan.

Schütze, U. (2015). Spacing techniques in second language vocabulary acquisition: short-term gains vs. long-term memory. *Language Teaching Research*, 19(1), 28–42.

Schütze, U., and Weimer-Stuckmann, G. (2010). Virtual vocabulary: research and learning in lexical processing. *CALICO Journal*, 27, 517–28.

(2011). Retention in SLA processing. *CALICO Journal*, 28, 460–72.

Service, L. (1992) Phonology, working memory, and foreign-language learning. *Quarterly Journal of Experimental Psychology*, 45A, 21–50.

Shallice, T. and Warrington, E. K. (1970). Independent functioning of verbal memory stores: a neuropsychological study. *Quarterly Journal of Experimental Psychology*, 22, 261–73.

Singer, W. (2006). *Vom Gehirn zum Bewußtsein. [From Mind to Consciousness.]* Frankfurt am Main: Suhrkamp.

Singleton, D. (1995). Introduction: a critical look at the Critical Period Hypothesis in second language acquisition research. In D. Singleton and Z. Lengyel (eds.), *The Age Factor in Second Language Acquisition: A Critical Look at the Critical Period Hypothesis* (pp. 1–29). Clevedon: Multilingual Matters.

(2007). The Critical Period Hypothesis: some problems. *Interlingüística*, 17, 48–56.

Skehan, P. (1998). *A Cognitive Approach to Language Learning*. Oxford University Press.

(2009a). Modeling second language performance: integrating complexity, accuracy, fluency, and lexis. *Applied Linguistics* 30, 510–32.

(2009b). Lexical performance by native and non-native speakers on language learning tasks. In B. Richards, H. M. Daller, D. Malvern, P. Meara, J. Milton, and J. Treffers-Daller (eds), *Vocabulary Studies in First and Second Language Acquisition: The Interface between Theory and Application* (pp. 107–24). Basingstoke: Palgrave Macmillan.

(2012). *Researching Tasks: Performance, Assessment, Pedagogy*. Shanghai: Shanghai Foreign Language Education Press/Amsterdam: De Gruyter.

Skehan, P., and Foster, P. (1997). Task type and processing conditions as influences on foreign language performance. *Language Teaching Research*, 1(3), 185–211.

(1999). The influence of task structure and processing conditions on narrative retellings. *Language Learning*, 49(1), 93–120.

(2001). Cognition and tasks. In P. Robinson (ed.), *Cognition and Second Language Learning* (pp. 183–205). New York: Cambridge University Press.

Sokoloff, L., Wechsler, R. L., Mangold, R., Balls, K., and Kety, S. S. (1953). Cerebral blood flow and oxygen consumption in hyperthyroidism before and after treatment. *Journal of Clinical Investigation*, 32, 202–08.

Speciale, G., Ellis, N., and Bywater, T. (2004). Phonological sequence learning and short-term store capacity determine second language vocabulary acquisition. *Applied Psycholinguistics*, 25(2), 293–321.

Spencer, J. P., Clearfield, M., Corbetta, D., Ulrich, B., Buchanan, P., and Schöner, G. (2006). Moving toward a grand theory of development: in memory of Esther Thelen. *Child Development*, 77, 1521–38.

Spivey, M. (2008). *The Continuity of Mind*. Oxford University Press.

Stemmer, B. (2010). A cognitive neuroscience perspective on learning and memory in aging. *Zeitschrift für Interkulturellen Fremdsprachenunterricht*, 15(1), 7–25. Available at http://zif.spz.tu-darmstadt.de/

Szagun. G. (1996). *Sprachentwicklung beim Kind*, 6th ed. Weinheim: Beltz.

Tager-Flusberg, H. (2001). Putting words together. In J. B. Gleason (ed.), *The Development of Language* (pp. 148–90). Boston: Pearson, Allyn and Bacon.

Thelen, E. (2005). Dynamic systems theory and the complexity of change. *Psychoanalytic Dialogues*, 15, 255–83.

Thomas, R. M. (2001). Connectionism and dynamic systems. In *Recent Theories of Human Development*. Thousand Oaks, CA: Sage.

Tranel, D., and Damasio, A. R. (2002). Neurobiological foundations of human memory. In A. D. Baddeley, M. D. Koppelman, and B. A. Wilson (eds.), *Handbook of Memory Disorders* (2nd ed., pp. 17–56). Chichester: Wiley.

Tranel, D., Damasio, H., and Damasio, A. R. (2000). Amnesia caused by herpes simplex encephalitis, infarctions in basal forebrain, and anoxia/ischemia. In F. Boller and J. Grafman (eds.), *Handbook of Neuropsychology* (2nd ed., pp. 85–110). Amsterdam: Elsevier Science.

Trojano, L, Stanzione, M., and Grossi, D. (1992). Short-term memory and verbal learning with auditory phonological coding defect: a neuropsychological case study. *Brain & Cognition*, 18, 12–33.

Tschichold, C. (2012). French vocabulary in Encore Tricolore: do pupils have a chance? *Language Learning Journal*, 40(1), 7–19.

Turvey, M. T., Brick, P., and Osborne, J. (1970). Proactive interference in short-term memory as a function of prior-item retention interval. *Quarterly Journal of Experimental Psychology*, 22, 142–47.

Vallar, G., and Baddeley, A. D. (1984). Fractionation of working memory: neuropsychological evidence for a phonological short-term store. *Journal of Verbal Learning and Verbal Behaviour*, 23, 151–61.

Vallar, G., and Papagno, C. (1993). Preserved vocabulary acquisition in Down's syndrome: the role of phonological short-term memory. *Cortex*, 29, 467–83.

(2002). Neuropsychological impairments of verbal short-term memory. In A. D. Baddeley, M. D. Kopelman, and B. A. Wilson (eds.), *Handbook of Memory Disorders* (2nd ed., pp. 249–70). Chichester: Wiley.

van Geert, P. (1991). A dynamic systems theory model of cognitive and language growth. *Psychological Review*, 98, 3–53.

(2008). The dynamic systems approach in the study of L1 and L2 acquisition: an introduction. *Modern Language Journal*, 92(2), 179–99.

Wagner, A., Maril, A., and Schacter, D. (2000). Interactions between forms of memory: when priming hinders new learning. *Journal of Cognitive Neuroscience*, 12, 52–60.

Wagner, A., Schacter, D., Rotte, M., Koutstaal, W., Maril, A., Dale, A., Rosen, B., and Buckner, R. (1998). Building memories: remembering and forgetting of verbal experiences as predicted by brain activity. *Science*, 281, 1188–91.

Wartenburger, I., Heekeren, H. R., Abutalebi, J., Cappa, S. F., Villringer, A., and Perani, D. (2003). Early setting of grammatical processing in the bilingual brain. *Neuron*, 37, 159–70.

Webb, S. (2005). Receptive and productive vocabulary learning: the effects of reading and writing on word knowledge. *Studies in Second Language Acquisition*, 27, 33–52.

Wilhelm, I., Diekelmann, S., Molzow, I., Ayoub, A., Mölle, M., and Born, J. (2011). Sleep selectively enhances memory expected to be of future relevance. *Journal of Neuroscience*, 31(5), 1563–69.

Willms, J., Shapiro, K., Peelen, M., Pajtas, P., Costa, A., Moo, L., and Caramazza, A. (2011). Language-invariant verb processing regions in Spanish-English bilinguals. *Neuroimage*, 57(1), 251–61.

Wilson, B. A., Baddeley, A., Evans, J., and Shiel, A. (1994). Errorless learning in the rehabilitation of memory impaired people. *Neuropsychological Rehabilitation*, 4, 307–26.

Wong, W., and Pyun, D. O. (2012). The effects of sentence writing on second language French and Korean lexical retention. *Canadian Modern Language Review*, 68(2), 164–89.

Zimmerman, C. B. (2009). *Word Knowledge: A Vocabulary Teacher's Handbook*. Oxford University Press.

Index